Cardiac Electrophysiology: Clinical Advances and Practice Updates

Cardiac Electrophysiology: Clinical Advances and Practice Updates

Editor

Ibrahim Marai

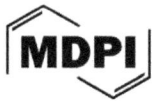

Basel • Beijing • Wuhan • Barcelona • Belgrade • Novi Sad • Cluj • Manchester

Editor
Ibrahim Marai
The Lydia and Carol Kittner,
Lea and Benjamin Davidai
Division of Cardiovascular
Medicine and Surgery, Tzafon
Medical Center
Poriya
Israel

Editorial Office
MDPI
St. Alban-Anlage 66
4052 Basel, Switzerland

This is a reprint of articles from the Special Issue published online in the open access journal *Journal of Clinical Medicine* (ISSN 2077-0383) (available at: https://www.mdpi.com/journal/jcm/special_issues/8X8K3QLO69).

For citation purposes, cite each article independently as indicated on the article page online and as indicated below:

Lastname, A.A.; Lastname, B.B. Article Title. *Journal Name* **Year**, *Volume Number*, Page Range.

ISBN 978-3-7258-0927-1 (Hbk)
ISBN 978-3-7258-0928-8 (PDF)
doi.org/10.3390/books978-3-7258-0928-8

© 2024 by the authors. Articles in this book are Open Access and distributed under the Creative Commons Attribution (CC BY) license. The book as a whole is distributed by MDPI under the terms and conditions of the Creative Commons Attribution-NonCommercial-NoDerivs (CC BY-NC-ND) license.

Contents

Michele Bertelli, Sebastiano Toniolo, Matteo Ziacchi, Alessio Gasperetti, Marco Schiavone, Roberto Arosio, et al.
Is Less Always More? A Prospective Two-Centre Study Addressing Clinical Outcomes in Leadless versus Transvenous Single-Chamber Pacemaker Recipients
Reprinted from: *Journal of Clinical Medicine* 2023, 11, 6071, doi:10.3390/jcm11206071 1

Shir Ben Asher Kestin, Ariel Israel, Eran Leshem, Anat Milman, Avi Sabbag, Ilan Goldengerg, et al.
Can the Norton Scale Score Be Used as an Adjunct Tool for Implantable Defibrillator Patient Selection? A Retrospective Single-Center Cohort Study
Reprinted from: *Journal of Clinical Medicine* 2023, 12, 214, doi:10.3390/jcm12010214 12

Ibrahim Marai, Rabea Haddad, Nizar Andria, Wadi Kinany, Yevgeni Hazanov, Bruce M. Kleinberg, et al.
Left Ventricular "Longitudinal Rotation" and Conduction Abnormalities—A New Outlook on Dyssynchrony
Reprinted from: *Journal of Clinical Medicine* 2023, 12, 745, doi:10.3390/jcm12030745 23

Moshe Katz, Amit Meitus, Michael Arad, Anthony Aizer, Eyal Nof and Roy Beinart
Long-Term Outcomes of Tachycardia-Induced Cardiomyopathy Compared with Idiopathic Dilated Cardiomyopathy
Reprinted from: *Journal of Clinical Medicine* 2023, 12, 1412, doi:10.3390/jcm12041412 34

Jan Berg, Alberto Preda, Nicolai Fierro, Alessandra Marzi, Andrea Radinovic, Paolo Della Bella, et al.
A Referral Center Experience with Cerebral Protection Devices: Challenging Cardiac Thrombus in the EP Lab
Reprinted from: *Journal of Clinical Medicine* 2023, 12, 1549, doi:10.3390/jcm12041549 48

Johnatan Nissan, Avi Sabbag, Roy Beinart and Eyal Nof
Inducibility of Multiple Ventricular Tachycardia's during a Successful Ablation Procedure Is a Marker of Ventricular Tachycardia Recurrence
Reprinted from: *Journal of Clinical Medicine* 2023, 12, 3660, doi:10.3390/jcm12113660 58

Anat Milman, Anat Wieder-Finesod, Guy Zahavi, Amit Meitus, Saar Kariv, Yuval Shafir, et al.
Complicated Pocket Infection in Patients Undergoing Lead Extraction: Characteristics and Outcomes
Reprinted from: *Journal of Clinical Medicine* 2023, 12, 4397, doi:10.3390/jcm12134397 67

Dicky A. Hanafy, Amiliana M. Soesanto, Budhi Setianto, Suzanna Immanuel, Sunu B. Raharjo, Herqutanto, et al.
Identification of Pacemaker Lead Position Using Fluoroscopy to Avoid Significant Tricuspid Regurgitation
Reprinted from: *Journal of Clinical Medicine* 2023, 12, 4782, doi:10.3390/jcm12144782 80

Botond Bocz, Dorottya Debreceni, Kristof-Ferenc Janosi, Marton Turcsan, Tamas Simor and Peter Kupo
Electroanatomical Mapping System-Guided vs. Intracardiac Echocardiography-Guided Slow Pathway Ablation: A Randomized, Single-Center Trial
Reprinted from: *Journal of Clinical Medicine* 2023, 12, 5577, doi:10.3390/jcm12175577 92

Marton Turcsan, Kristof-Ferenc Janosi, Dorottya Debreceni, Daniel Toth, Botond Bocz, Tamas Simor, et al.
Intracardiac Echocardiography Guidance Improves Procedural Outcomes in Patients Undergoing Cavotricuspidal Isthmus Ablation for Typical Atrial Flutter
Reprinted from: *Journal of Clinical Medicine* **2023**, *12*, 6277, doi:10.3390/jcm12196277 . . . . **101**

Marta Telishevska, Sarah Lengauer, Tilko Reents, Verena Kantenwein, Miruna Popa, Fabian Bahlke, et al.
Long-Term Follow-Up of Empirical Slow Pathway Ablation in Pediatric and Adult Patients with Suspected AV Nodal Reentrant Tachycardia
Reprinted from: *Journal of Clinical Medicine* **2023**, *12*, 6532, doi:10.3390/jcm12206532 . . . . **110**

Shmuel Tiosano, Ariel Banai, Wesam Mulla, Ido Goldenberg, Gabriella Bayshtok, Uri Amit, et al.
Left Atrial Appendage Occlusion versus Novel Oral Anticoagulation for Stroke Prevention in Atrial Fibrillation—One-Year Survival
Reprinted from: *Journal of Clinical Medicine* **2023**, *12*, 6693, doi:10.3390/jcm12206693 . . . . **121**

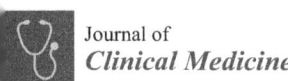

Article

Is Less Always More? A Prospective Two-Centre Study Addressing Clinical Outcomes in Leadless versus Transvenous Single-Chamber Pacemaker Recipients

Michele Bertelli [1,†], Sebastiano Toniolo [1,†], Matteo Ziacchi [1,*], Alessio Gasperetti [2], Marco Schiavone [2], Roberto Arosio [2], Claudio Capobianco [1], Gianfranco Mitacchione [2], Giovanni Statuto [1], Andrea Angeletti [1], Cristian Martignani [1], Igor Diemberger [1], Giovanni Battista Forleo [2] and Mauro Biffi [1]

1 IRCCS Azienda Ospedaliero, Universitaria di Bologna, 40122 Bologna, Italy
2 Unità Operativa di Cardiologia, ASST-Fatebenefratelli-Sacco, Ospedale Luigi Sacco University, 20157 Milano, Italy
* Correspondence: matteo.ziacchi@gmail.com; Tel.: +39-051-2143598
† These authors contributed equally to this work.

Abstract: (1) Background: Leadless (LL) stimulation is perceived to lower surgical, vascular, and lead-related complications compared to transvenous (TV) pacemakers, yet controlled studies are lacking and real-life experience is non-conclusive. (2) Aim: To prospectively analyse survival and complication rates in leadless versus transvenous VVIR pacemakers. (3) Methods: Prospective analysis of mortality and complications in 344 consecutive VVIR TV and LL pacemaker recipients between June 2015 and May 2021. Indications for VVIR pacing were "slow" AF, atrio-ventricular block in AF or in sinus rhythm in bedridden cognitively impaired patients. LL indication was based on individualised clinical judgement. (4) Results: 72 patients received LL and 272 TV VVIR pacemakers. LL pacemaker indications included ongoing/expected chronic haemodialysis, superior venous access issues, active lifestyle with low pacing percentage expected, frailty causing high bleeding/infectious risk, previous valvular endocarditis, or device infection requiring extraction. No significant difference in the overall acute and long-term complication rate was observed between LL and TV cohorts, with greater mortality occurring in TV due to selection of older patients. (5) Conclusions: Given the low complication rate and life expectancy in this contemporary VVIR cohort, extending LL indications to all VVIR candidates is unlikely to provide clear-cut benefits. Considering the higher costs of LL technology, careful patient selection is mandatory for LL PMs to become advantageous, i.e., in the presence of vascular access issues, high bleeding/infectious risk, and long life expectancy, rendering lead-related issues and repeated surgery relevant in the long-term perspective.

Keywords: VVIR pacemaker; leadless pacemaker; patient selection; complications; clinical outcome

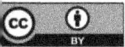

1. Introduction

Single-chamber VVIR pacing constitutes the mainstay treatment of atrio-ventricular block in the presence of atrial fibrillation (AF), representing 10–15% of all pacemaker (PM) implants in Western countries [1]. VVIR candidates are typically older and with more comorbidities, thus having a lower life-expectancy than their dual-chamber counterparts [2]. Implanting an intravascular lead and creating a subcutaneous pocket is still burdened by a number of potential short- and long-term complications, namely, bleeding, infection, and pneumothorax, which increase in incidence and morbidity with patient age [3]. The introduction of leadless (LL) PMs, delivered via transfemoral venous route, appeared to address these issues by providing right-ventricular (RV) stimulation without the need for an intravascular lead or a subcutaneous pocket [4]. While safety and efficacy profiles of LL technology have been characterised in previous studies [5–7], it is still unclear whether its application to all VVIR candidates does provide a substantial complication- and survival-related advantage compared to its transvenous (TV) counterpart. To date, no randomised trial comparing LL and TV VVIR outcomes has been conducted, with clinical evidence being limited to prospective or retrospective studies. Furthermore, earlier studies have based their comparison on historical TV cohorts associated with higher complication rates than contemporary ones, thereby likely overestimating any benefit from LL PMs [5,6]. Indeed, the TV PM safety profile is continuously improving, owing to awareness of best practice recommendations and standardisation of training [8–10]. This is reflected by more recent LL studies comparing outcomes with contemporary TV VVIR cohorts, which overall failed to demonstrate a clearcut advantage in LL patients [7,11], and applies also to the large comparative analysis of TV and LL outcomes obtained from the Medicare database over a 2-year follow-up period (6219 LL vs. 10,212 TV patients) [12,13]. While demonstrating lower rates of reintervention and overall complications (albeit higher rates of pericardial effusion) in LL PMs, the study failed to demonstrate any difference in 30-day and 2-year all-cause mortality [12]. As a result, current evidence points to a rather mixed picture concerning complication and survival benefits in LL compared to traditional TV VVIR PMs. Owing to the limited life expectancy of VVIR recipients and to the time-dependent increase of lead-related issues [3,14], it can be argued that the majority of VVIR candidates are unlikely to have sufficient life expectancy to be negatively impacted by lead- or pocket-related risks. Given the significantly higher costs of leadless technology (10 times a TV system in our country), a real-world prospective assessment of the true scope of VVIR LL application in current clinical practice is needed. For these reasons, we aimed to observe whether utilisation of TV and LL based on clinical judgement would prove clinically effective in minimising overall complications in VVIR PM recipients.

2. Materials and Methods

This is a prospective study of 344 consecutive patients undergoing either LL (Micra™, Medtronic Inc., Minneapolis, MN, USA) or TV VVIR pacemaker implantation in two tertiary cardiology centres in Italy between June 2015 (Micra™ market release in Italy) and May 2021. We planned this observational study at the beginning of our experience with LL systems on all consecutive VVIR recipients at our centres. Indications for VVIR pacing included "slow conducted" AF, atrio-ventricular block with comorbid AF (either permanent or accepted as "destination rhythm") or, in a minority of cases, with sinus rhythm in bedridden cognitively impaired patients. Assignment to either LL or TV group was based on clinical judgement. In particular, LL was favoured in the presence of ongoing or expected chronic haemodialysis, superior venous access issues such as occlusion or need for its preservation, active lifestyle with low amount of pacing expected, frailty causing high bleeding and infectious risk (defined as at least 2 amongst: combined anticoagulation and antiplatelet therapy that could not be interrupted due to high thromboembolic risk, ongoing long-term steroid therapy, ongoing chemotherapy, BMI < 18.5 kg/m^2), valvular endocarditis or implantable electronic device infection treated by lead extraction within the previous 6 months.

Lead insertion in TV was performed either via cephalic vein cutdown or subclavian/axillary vein puncture. The latter occurred at operator's discretion, blinded or under fluoroscopic guidance. TV leads were placed either in the RV apex or septum at the operator's preference and position was confirmed by right/left anterior oblique, or latero-lateral radiographic views as per EHRA expert consensus guidelines (8). LL devices, in turn, were deployed via transfemoral vein route following the manufacturer's recommendations with vein closure achieved by purse-string suture followed by 5-min manual compression.

Anticoagulation therapy was not interrupted in any patient unless dictated by specific clinical indications. Specifically, vitamin K antagonists were tapered to the INR range of 2–2.5 for the week following device implantation in patients with CHA2DS2-VASc score ≤ 3. Direct oral anticoagulants (DOAC) were held on the day of implantation and resumed 24 h thereafter. Dual antiplatelet therapy was not interrupted. Suction drains were used in TV recipients to prevent pocket haematoma in case of dual antiplatelet, anticoagulant plus antiplatelet therapy, incomplete haemostasis, or unstable/high (>2.5) INR, and removed at bleeding cessation on desired antithrombotic regimen (usually within 48–72 h).

As per local protocol, antibiotic prophylaxis consisted of 2 g cefazolin or 1200 mg clindamycin, in penicillin allergic patients, 30 min prior to skin incision. In patients with hospitalisation duration greater than 7 days, 1–2 g vancomycin (dose adjusted to renal function) was used 90–120 min prior to skin incision. In patients with suction drain, in turn, prophylaxis was continued until drain removal. None of the TV patients received a TYRX™ antibiotic envelope.

Device and wound status were assessed 2–3 weeks after hospital discharge. Subsequently, clinical follow-up was performed at 6 months and twice yearly thereafter, compiling data on patient status and pacemaker performance. Stimulation percentage was weighed against time elapsed between device interrogations. Clinical information, including incurring medical events related to comorbidities and death, was obtained during subsequent hospital admissions, ambulatory visits, remote patient follow-up, or by consulting regional telematic databases (in patients unable to attend ambulatory visits).

Data from the TV and LL cohorts were analysed with IBM SPSS Statistics (26.0 version for Windows; IBM Corp; Armonk, NY, USA). Variable distribution was assessed using the Shapiro–Wilks test. Continuous variables were then evaluated with the Mann–Whitney U test for non-parametric data, while the Kruskal–Wallis test was used when comparing more than two groups. Categorical variables, in turn, were compared with Chi-square tests of independence between groups. Thereafter, survival analyses for both all-cause and cardiovascular mortality were conducted using Kaplan–Meier plots and the log-rank test. Multivariate analyses of all-cause mortality were performed using Cox regression. The level of statistical significance for all the above was set at $p < 0.05$.

3. Results

3.1. Baseline Characteristics

Seventy-two patients (20.9%) received LL and 272 (79.1%) TV VVIR pacemakers (Table 1). Patients in the LL group were significantly younger than in the TV group (median age 79.5 ± 2.5 vs. 85.0 ± 1.0), with diabetes and ongoing haemodialysis being more prevalent (26.4 vs. 18.0% and 6.9 vs. 0.7%, respectively), while chronic kidney disease (GFR < 60 mL/min/1.73 m^2) was more common in the TV group (57.7 vs. 36.1%), as reported in Table 1. Atrial fibrillation, either permanent or paroxysmal, was significantly more frequent in the TV group (96.3 vs. 80.6%). No other significant difference in comorbidities (i.e., hypertension, ischaemic heart disease, left ventricular ejection fraction, history of percutaneous or surgical treatment of valvular heart disease) was observed between groups (Table 1). Amongst the 72 LL recipients, five (6.9%) were on haemodialysis, eight (11.1%) had a completely occluded subclavian vein while seven (9.7%) needed superior vein patency maintenance, 16 (22.2%) were active patients with only sporadic pacing required to prevent long pauses, 17 (23.6%) were frail based on the aforementioned criteria, two (2.8%) had recent surgery due to valvular endocarditis, and four (5.6%) had undergone CIED extraction because of pocket or endovascular CIED infection.

3.2. Procedural Data

Both procedural and fluoroscopy times were significantly longer in LL compared to TV patients (median procedural time 74 ± 13 vs. 55 ± 5 min, $p < 0.01$; median fluoroscopy time 8.4 ± 2.3 vs. 3.0 ± 1.0 min, $p < 0.01$). In the LL group, most implants occurred in the interventricular septum (88.9%) and only a minority (11.1%) in the right ventricular apex. In the TV group, in turn, the majority of implants were either in the right ventricular apex (50.7%) or interventricular septum (42.7%), with only some in the His bundle (4.8%), right ventricular outflow tract (0.4%), or left ventricle via a coronary vein (1.1%). Fluoroscopy times were not different for septal or apical implants in either group (Figure 1). In terms of electrical parameters at implantation, no statistically significant difference was observed between LL and TV groups in mean capture threshold (0.75 ± 0.08 V vs. 0.69 ± 0.04 V), impedance (748 ± 28 vs. 698 ± 15 Ohm), and mean intrinsic R wave amplitude (9.8 ± 0.6 vs. 10.8 ± 0.4 mV) (Table 2).

Table 1. Baseline patient characteristics and 30-day perioperative complications in LL and TV PM recipients.

	Leadless (n = 72)	Transvenous (n = 272)	Significance ($p < 0.05$)
Baseline characteristics			
Age; median [SEM *]	79.5 [2.5]	85.0 [1.0]	$p < 0.01$
Sex (female)	26/72 (36%)	111/272 (41%)	$p = 0.47$
Diabetes mellitus	19/72 (26.4%)	49/272 (18.0%)	$p < 0.01$
Hypertension	51/72 (70.8%)	212/272 (77.9%)	$p = 0.21$
Ejection fraction; median [SEM]	57 [3]%	59 [2]%	$p = 0.49$
Permanent atrial fibrillation	58/72 (80.6%)	262/272 (96.3%)	$p < 0.01$
Ischaemic heart disease	14/72 (19.4%)	83/272 (30.5%)	$p = 0.06$
Previous CIED extraction	7/72 (9.7%)	2/272 (0.7%)	$p < 0.01$
Surgical or percutaneous treatment of valvular disease	20/72 (27.8%)	82/272 (30.1%)	$p = 0.70$
Chronic kidney disease ** (GFR < 60 mL/min/1.73 m^2)	26/72 (36.1%)	157/272 (57.7%)	$p < 0.01$
Chronic haemodialysis	5/72 (6.9%)	2/272 (0.7%)	$p < 0.01$
Bedridden/cognitive impairment	0/72 (0%)	3/272 (1.1%)	$p = 0.37$
30-day perioperative complications			
Pericardial effusion	0/72 (0%)	4/272 (1.5%)	$p = 0.30$
Tamponade	0/72 (0%)	1/272 (0.4%)	$p = 0.61$
Lead/device dislocation	1/72 (1.4%)	0/272 (0%)	$p = 0.06$
Pneumothorax [requiring drainage]	/	6/272 (2.2%) [1/272 (0.4%)]	/
Haematoma [requiring surgical revision]	3/72 (4.2%) [0/72 (0%)]	3/272 (1.1%) [1/272 (0.4%)]	$p = 0.08$
Overall	4/72 (5.6%)	14/272 (5.1%)	$p = 0.33$

* SEM: standard error of the median; ** eGFR < 60 mL/min/1.73 m^2.

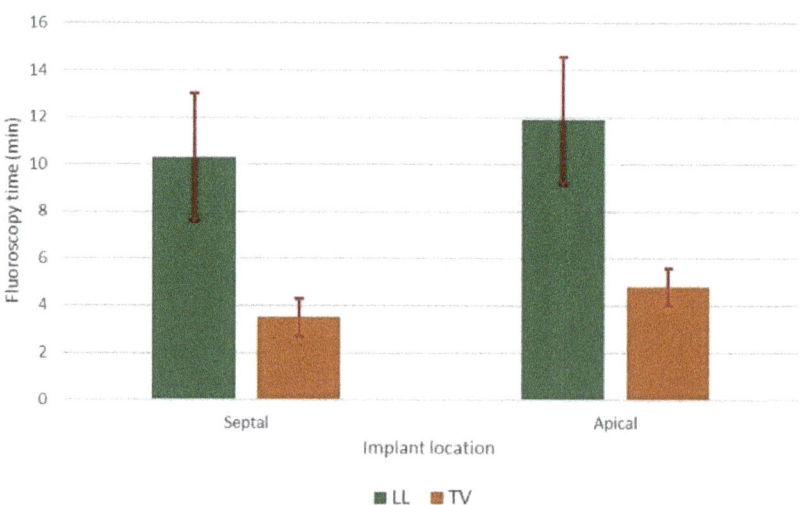

Figure 1. Fluoroscopy times in septal vs. apical implants for LL and TV PMs.

Table 2. Electrical parameters after implantation and patient data/electrical parameters at follow-up.

	Leadless (n = 72)	Transvenous (n = 272)	Significance ($p < 0.05$)
Electrical parameters after implantation			
Mean capture threshold (V × 0.4 ms)	0.75 ± 0.08	0.69 ± 0.04	$p = 0.79$
Mean impedance (Ohm)	748 ± 28	698 ± 15	$p = 0.06$
Mean intrinsic R wave amplitude (mV)	9.8 ± 0.6	10.8 ± 0.4	$p = 0.58$
Electrical parameters at follow-up			
Mean capture threshold (V × 0.4 ms)	0.62 ± 0.04	0.79 ± 0.03	**$p = 0.005$**
Mean capture threshold increase > 1 V	2/72 (2.7%)	9/262 (3.4%)	$p = 0.12$
Mean impedance (Ohm)	636 ± 18	606 ± 14	**$p = 0.009$**
Mean intrinsic R wave amplitude (mV)	11.6 ± 0.5	12.0 ± 0.4	$p = 0.86$
Patient data at follow-up			
Mean follow-up time (months)	22.8 ± 2.6	23.7 ± 1.1	$p = 0.31$
Superficial Suture Infection [requiring surgical revision]	0/72 (0%)	3/272 (1.1%) [2/272 (0.8%)]	$p = 0.37$
Haematoma	0/72 (0%)	1/272 (0.4%)	$p = 0.61$
Skin sore	0/72 (0%)	1/272 (0.4%)	$p = 0.61$
Overall long-term complications	0/72 (0%)	5/272 (1.9%)	$p = 0.25$
Pacing system revisions [Repositioning] [Lead addition]	0/72 (0%)	6/272 (2.3%) [5/272 (1.9%)] [1/272 (0.4%)]	$p = 0.20$

3.3. Data at Follow-Up

Mean follow-up times for LL and TV groups were comparable (22.8 ± 2.6 months vs. 23.7 ± 1.1 months, $p = 0.31$). Overall, no LL patients required pacing system revision while six patients (2.2%) in the TV groups required either lead repositioning (five cases) or addition (one case) because of a high pacing threshold. Both groups demonstrated stability of electrical parameters, with only nine patients in the TV group (3.4%) and two in the LL group (2.7%) having an increase greater than 1 V in capture threshold (Table 2).

3.4. Complication Analysis

On analysis of periprocedural and long-term complications, no significant difference in the individual and overall complication rate over the entire follow-up period was observed between LL and TV groups (overall acute complications: 5.6 vs. 5.1%, $p = 0.33$; overall long-term complications: 0 vs. 1.9%, $p = 0.25$). The three groin haematomas occurring in the LL group involved one patient on DOAC (apixaban) and two patients on warfarin (pre-procedural INR 2.3 and 1.44, respectively). Regarding haematomas occurring in the TV population, one occurred in a patient on rivaroxaban and aspirin, and in two cases in patients on warfarin with pre-procedural INR 2.29 and 2, respectively, the latter being the only case requiring surgical revision. Overall, six pneumothoraces (2.2%) occurred in the TV group, when performing either blinded puncture of the subclavian vein (three cases) or under fluoroscopic guidance in the postero-anterior (PA) view (three cases). Of the latter, one occurred after crossing to the contralateral side because of an occluded subclavian vein. Only one out of six pneumothoraces required drainage. No pneumothorax occurred in the 68 patients whose vein access was obtained via the cephalic vein or by axillary puncture under 35°-caudal-tilt fluoroscopic guidance in PA view. Four TV PM recipients had mild pericardial effusion at hospital discharge, lead placement being in all these cases in the right ventricular apex; in two of these, no echocardiogram was available in the 2 weeks before implant, thus raising uncertainty on the true correlation with the procedure. The single case of tamponade occurred because of inadvertent RV free wall placement while aiming at the interventricular septum; no long-term sequelae occurred to this patient. Lastly, the single episode of dislocation in the LL group occurred in a patient during device placement in the right ventricular apex, as the 18th consecutive case of the most experienced operator: multiple deployments (>6) were attempted because of thrombus formation at the cup of the delivery catheter preventing ventricular capture at threshold measurements. When capture was eventually obtained, anchoring was stable on two tines only. As a result, the Micra unit dislodged and was retrieved by means of a 2-snares technique to turn it straight as to enter the large-bore sheath (Supplementary Material online). At follow-up, no LL patient, but six patients in the TV group, underwent lead repositioning (five cases) or lead addition (one case) because of a pacing threshold increase above 2V@04ms to maximise pacemaker longevity.

3.5. Mortality and Multivariate Analysis

By Kaplan–Meyer survival analysis, TV recipients had greater all-cause and cardiovascular mortality (Figure 2). Patients from both the LL and TV group were stratified based on stimulation percentage as assessed during device interrogation at last follow-up. Non-cardiovascular as well as cardiovascular mortality were then plotted across five quintiles of stimulation percentage in both groups (Figure 3). On multivariate analysis of mortality in TV and LL cohorts, only age in the TV group appeared to significantly impact mortality. Similarly, on analysis of the entire population only age displayed a significant association with mortality (Table 3).

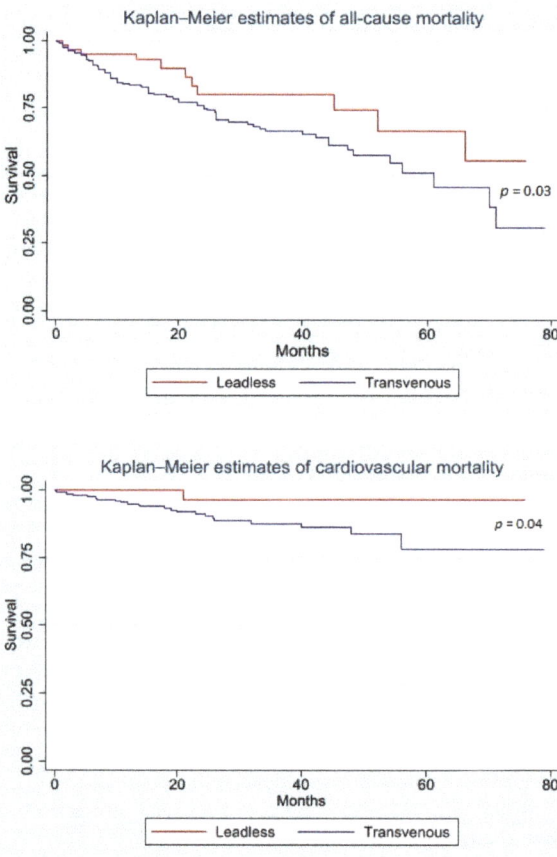

Figure 2. Kaplan–Meyer estimates of all-cause and cardiovascular mortality in LL and TV PM recipients over the follow-up period.

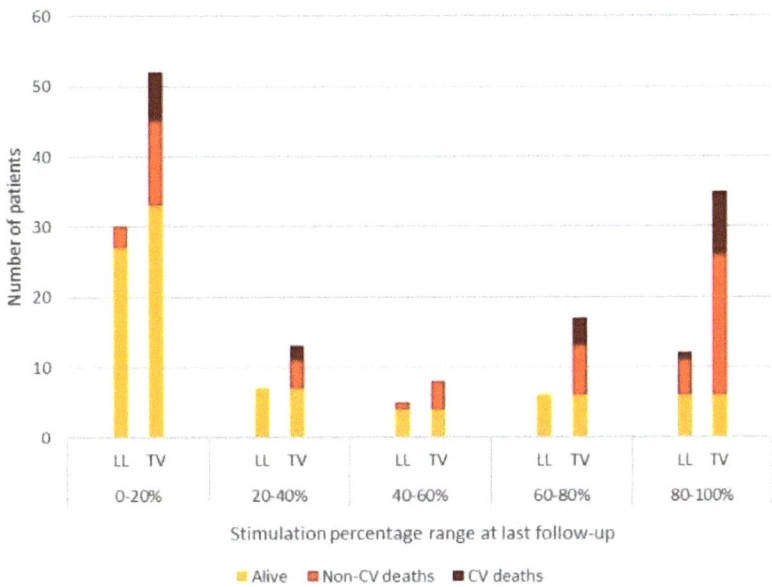

Figure 3. Cardiovascular and non-cardiovascular mortality in LL and TV PM recipients weighed against stimulation percentage at last follow-up.

Table 3. Multivariate analysis of all-cause mortality in LL and TV cohorts and on the entire population.

Multivariate Analysis of All-Cause Mortality in LL vs. TV					
Variable	Leadless (n = 72) Hazard Ratio [95% CI]	p Value		Transvenous (n = 272) Hazard Ratio [95% CI]	p Value
Age	1.019 [0.909–1.142]	0.74		1.073 [1.026–1.122]	0.002
Female sex	1.381 [0.227–8.394]	0.73		1.507 [0.881–2.576]	0.13
Diabetes mellitus	1.352 [0.1666–11.037]	0.78		1.864 [1.020–3.406]	0.05
Chronic kidney disease *	0.564 [0.078–4.069]	0.57		1.774 [0.922–3.413]	0.09
Ischaemic heart disease	2.109 [0.421–10.550]	0.36		1.156 [0.666–2.005]	0.61
Left ventricular ejection fraction	0.958 [0.878–1.045]	0.33		1.000 [0.974–1.027]	1.00
Ventricular stimulation percentage	5.856 [0.994–34.484]	0.05		1.128 [0.655–1.943]	0.66
Multivariate Analysis of All-Cause Mortality in Both Cohorts					
Variable	Hazard Ratio [95% CI]			p Value	
Leadless vs. transvenous	0.929 [0.422–2.043]			0.85	
Age	1.071 [1.027–1.117]			0.001	
Female sex	1.473 [0.888–2.444]			0.13	
Diabetes mellitus	1.617 [0.911–2.869]			0.10	
Chronic kidney disease *	1.704 [0.953–3.047]			0.07	
Ischaemic heart disease	1.226 [0.741–2.031]			0.43	
Left ventricular ejection fraction	0.995 [0.971–1.019]			0.67	
Percentage ventricular stimulation	1.347 [0.805–2.253]			0.26	

* eGFR < 60 mL/min/1.73 m^2.

4. Discussion

From this dual centre prospective study, a number of conclusions can be drawn on the current clinical application of leadless versus transvenous pacemakers in the setting of VVIR pacing. Given the lack of evidence from randomised trials on LL and TV outcomes, pacing system selection in this study was based on the principle of individualised therapy and resulted in similar complication rates in the two arms. Another important observation is that mortality of VVIR recipients is such that exposure to lead-related unwanted events in TV recipients is negligible, thus likely blunting any expected advantage of LL technology. Factors such as lack of or necessity to spare thoracic veins for future intravenous therapy, high infectious or surgical risks (due to bleeding or lead-related complications) related to clinical frailty, and long-term exposure to implanted pacing system in patients with relatively long life expectancy and active lifestyle, were all considered to favour LL pacing. According to this pre-defined strategy, LL recipients were either those with a more challenging clinical profile or minimal probability of long-term pacing dependence. As a result, they were on average younger than their TV counterparts, which contributed to a lower mortality. A particularly relevant group were patients on permanent haemodialysis where a transvenous approach is often precluded by either superior vein occupation by indwelling catheters or need for their preservation for dialysis treatment, a setting where LL VVIR safety has been confirmed by a recent retrospective study [15].

In agreement with the current literature, our study confirms the low complication rate in TV VVIR recipients, with a substantial reduction relative to historical transvenous cohorts and with no significant difference compared to leadless recipients both in terms of perioperative and long-term complications. Indeed, a recent meta-analysis on four studies including TV control cohorts (344 LL vs. 400 TV patients in total) showed no difference in incidence of haematoma, pericardial effusion, device dislocation, any complication, and death between LL and TV PMs, with a 3.11% pooled complication rate [16]. Importantly, the latter figure, comparable to our study, corroborates the notion that contemporary TV complication rates are significantly lower than historical ones [6,17]. Similar findings also apply to another recent meta-analysis where lower complication rates in the LL group were observed only when compared with historical TV cohorts, while analysis of studies with contemporary TV cohorts revealed a higher 1-year complication rate in LL VVIR recipients [18].

The improvement in TV outcomes over recent years is likely due to increasing efforts aimed at standardising implantation techniques as well as training programmes [8]. Indeed, one of the main challenges of comparing outcomes in LL and TV VVIR PMs lies in the different learning pathways of these two procedures. On the one hand, MicraTM release involved specific training of a limited number of very experienced implanters who would later provide guidance to further operators, with a consequent predictable learning curve, leading to declining complication rates between Investigational Device Exemption (IDE) and later real-world studies [5,6]. On the other hand, transvenous lead implantation has evolved over decades, with diversity in implantation techniques across implanters and thus greater challenges in procedural standardisation. Clear examples of the potential benefits of TV technique standardisation provided in our study are the absence of pneumothorax when adopting a 35° caudal tilt axillary puncture and, on the contrary, increasing risk of inadvertent RV perforation and tamponade when omitting radiologic confirmation of true septal lead placement. Only recently, practical recommendations on CIED surgery, vascular access, and lead placement have been published with the aim of maximising lead performance and minimising both short and long-term complications [8]. Given the limited standardising efforts conducted so far, these recommendations are expected to significantly impact clinicians' proficiency in the next few years. Examples of the potential benefits of such efforts, detailed in the EHRA expert consensus document, are avoidance of pneumothorax by widespread cephalic vein use or ultrasound-guided vein puncture (not used in this study), or minimisation of inadvertent RV free wall perforation risk by use of specific fluoroscopic views [8]. These simple behavioural changes have been shown to bring down TV complications to 1.5%, possibly impacting long-term outcomes as well. In further support of the dramatic impact that procedural standardisation can bring about, Ahsan et al. demonstrated that the application of a simple infection-control protocol was able to halve CIED infections [10].

An additional point of reflection is hinted at by the mortality analysis of our VVIR cohorts, confirming an extremely low life expectancy of VVIR candidates, mostly driven by non-cardiovascular causes. In keeping with our patient selection criteria, patients in the

LL cohort were younger and had thus a significantly longer life expectancy on average. In the setting of such limited life expectancy, long-term lead-related and infective risks, which are known to be time-dependent [14], are unlikely to be fully expressed and thus to have significant prognostic relevance, thereby undermining the most significant advantage of LL systems. From the data collected at follow-up, one of the advantages of LL devices appeared to be the lower, albeit not statistically significant, rate of reintervention. This observation, in line with a recent study by El-Chami et al. [12], highlights the importance of selecting patients with sufficient life expectancy to significantly benefit from a lower long-term reintervention rate in LL PMs. Nonetheless, lead-related reintervention needs to be considered in the correct perspective since these were performed to correct for high pacing thresholds, with a view to maximise device longevity. While the unanticipated increase of pacing threshold is well known in literature and lead manipulation is feasible in TV devices [19], it is not in LL pacers, and demands a new device implantation with far superior costs, suggesting a significant bias towards reintervention in TV compared to LL PMs. On further analysis of survival data, we found that a higher amount of stimulation identifies patients with limited life expectancy where long-term lead-related risks are likely negligible. This finding further corroborates our selection criterion whereby patients with expected pacing-dependence underwent TV implantation. Our study also confirms the excellent long-term electrical performance of LL devices. This information, together with recent work putting forward a number of predictors of poor LL electrical performance, suggest that LL long-term performance is not only highly efficient but has also a significant degree of predictability [20]. Lastly, our multivariate analysis on survival did not identify any significant factor associated with all-cause mortality at follow-up, with the exception of age, whose associated comorbidities pose a heavy burden of non-cardiovascular mortality (Table 3, Figures 2 and 3).

In summary, the main advantages of LL devices appear to lie in the decreased long-term reintervention rates, whereas benefits in terms of short-term complications appear far less clear-cut [6,9–12]. Our experience confirms the usefulness of our clinically-oriented implantation strategy when aiming for "individualised" therapy with a view to minimise both short- and long-term complications. Moreover, in the long-term perspective, the shortcomings of LL pacemakers, such as lack of physiologic ventricular activation as enabled by conduction system pacing, limited diagnostics, and absence of wireless remote patient monitoring, may be detrimental for patients' management [13].

5. Conclusions

Given the limited complication rates observed in this contemporary single-chamber TV cohort and low life expectancy of this population, extending LL indications to all VVIR recipients is unlikely to provide a clearcut clinical benefit to this particular patient group. Considering the higher costs of LL technology, these data prompt a careful selection of patients most likely to gain a real advantage from LL pacemakers. In addition to the setting of vascular access issues and high bleeding or infectious risk, these may include patients with sufficient life expectancy for lead issues and repeated surgery to become relevant in the long-term perspective.

Supplementary Materials: The following supporting information can be downloaded at: https://www.mdpi.com/article/10.3390/jcm11206071/s1, Video S1: Leadless pacemaker stability testing; Video S2: Dislodgement below the tricuspid valve; Video S3: Pacemaker dislodged into right atrium; Video S4: Retrieval of leadless device.

Author Contributions: Conceptualisation, M.B. (Mauro Biffi) and M.Z.; methodology, M.B. (Mauro Biffi) and M.Z.; validation, M.Z., G.M., G.B.F., I.D. and M.B. (Mauro Biffi); formal analysis, M.B. (Michele Bertelli); investigation, M.B. (Michele Bertelli), S.T., A.G., M.S., R.A., C.C., G.S., A.A., C.M., I.D.; data curation, M.B. (Michele Bertelli) and S.T.; writing—original draft preparation, M.B. (Michele Bertelli) and S.T.; writing—review and editing, M.B. (Michele Bertelli); supervision, M.B. (Mauro Biffi) and M.Z.; project administration, M.B. (Mauro Biffi) and M.Z. All authors have read and agreed to the published version of the manuscript.

Funding: This research received no external funding.

Institutional Review Board Statement: This study was conducted in accordance with the Declaration of Helsinki and approved by the Hospital Ethics Committee (10/2016/U/Oss).

Informed Consent Statement: All patients treated by leadless or transvenous pacemakers gave their written consent for participation in clinical trials or registries.

Conflicts of Interest: The authors declare no conflict of interest.

References

1. Proclemer, A.; Zecchin, M.; D'Onofrio, A.; Boriani, G.; Ricci, R.P.; Rebellato, L.; Ghidina, M.; Bianco, G.; Bernardelli, E.; Miconi, A.; et al. Registro Italiano Pacemaker e Defibrillatori—Bollettino Periodico 2018. Associazione Italiana di Aritmologia e Cardiostimolazione [The Pacemaker and Implantable Cardioverter-Defibrillator Registry of the Italian Association of Arrhythmology and Cardiac Pacing—2018 Annual report]. *G. Ital. Cardiol. (Rome)* **2020**, *21*, 157–169.
2. Biffi, M.; Capobianco, C.; Spadotto, A.; Bartoli, L.; Sorrentino, S.; Minguzzi, A.; Piemontese, G.P.; Angeletti, A.; Toniolo, S.; Statuto, G. Pacing devices to treat bradycardia: Current status and future perspectives. *Expert Rev. Med. Devices* **2021**, *18*, 161–177. [CrossRef] [PubMed]
3. Krahn, A.D.; Longtin, Y.; Philippon, F.; Birnie, D.H.; Manlucu, J.; Angaran, P.; Rinne, C.; Coutu, B.; Low, R.A.; Essebag, V.; et al. Prevention of Arrhythmia Device Infection Trial: The PADIT Trial. *J. Am. Coll. Cardiol.* **2018**, *72*, 3098–3109. [CrossRef]
4. Ritter, P.; Duray, G.Z.; Steinwender, C.; Soejima, K.; Omar, R.; Mont, L.; Boersma, L.V.; Knops, R.E.; Chinitz, L.; Zhang, S.; et al. Early performance of a miniaturized leadless cardiac pacemaker: The Micra Transcatheter Pacing Study. *Eur. Heart J.* **2015**, *36*, 2510–2519. [CrossRef] [PubMed]
5. Reynolds, D.; Duray, G.Z.; Omar, R.; Soejima, K.; Neuzil, P.; Zhang, S.; Narasimhan, C.; Steinwender, C.; Brugada, J.; Lloyd, M.; et al. A Leadless Intracardiac Transcatheter Pacing System. *N. Engl. J. Med.* **2016**, *374*, 533–541. [CrossRef]
6. El-Chami, M.F.; Al-Samadi, F.; Clementy, N.; Garweg, C.; Martinez-Sande, J.L.; Piccini, J.P.; Iacopino, S.; Lloyd, M.; Viñolas Prat, X.; Jacobsen, M.D.; et al. Updated performance of the Micra transcatheter pacemaker in the real-world setting: A comparison to the investigational study and a transvenous historical control. *Heart Rhythm.* **2018**, *15*, 1800–1807. [CrossRef] [PubMed]
7. Martinez-Sande, J.L.; Garcia-Seara, J.; Gonzalez-Melchor, L.; Rodriguez-Mañero, M.; Baluja, A.; Fernandez-Lopez, X.A.; Gonzalez Juanatey, J.R. Conventional single-chamber pacemakers versus transcatheter pacing systems in a «real world» cohort of patients: A comparative prospective single-center study. *Indian Pacing Electrophysiol. J.* **2021**, *21*, 89–94. [CrossRef]
8. Burri, H.; Starck, C.; Auricchio, A.; Biffi, M.; Burri, M.; D'Avila, A.; Deharo, J.C.; Glikson, M.; Israel, C.; Lau, C.P.; et al. EHRA expert consensus statement and practical guide on optimal implantation technique for conventional pacemakers and implantable cardioverter-defibrillators: Endorsed by the Heart Rhythm Society (HRS), the Asia Pacific Heart Rhythm Society (APHRS), and the Latin-American Heart Rhythm Society (LAHRS). *Europace* **2021**, *23*, 983–1008.
9. Mascheroni, J.; Mont, L.; Stockburger, M.; Patwala, A.; Retzlaff, H.; Gallagher, A.G. A validation study of intraoperative performance metrics for training novice cardiac resynchronization therapy implanters. *Int. J. Cardiol.* **2020**, *307*, 48–54. [CrossRef] [PubMed]
10. Ahsan, S.Y.; Saberwal, B.; Lambiase, P.D.; Koo, C.Y.; Lee, S.; Gopalamurugan, A.B.; Rogers, D.P.; Lowe, M.D.; Chow, A.W. A simple infection-control protocol to reduce serious cardiac device infections. *Europace* **2014**, *16*, 1482–1489. [CrossRef]
11. Piccini, J.P.; El-Chami, M.; Wherry, K.; Crossley, G.H.; Kowal, R.C.; Stromberg, K.; Longacre, C.; Hinnenthal, J.; Bockstedt, L. Contemporaneous Comparison of Outcomes Among Patients Implanted with a Leadless vs. Transvenous Single-Chamber Ventricular Pacemaker. *JAMA Cardiol.* **2021**, *6*, 1187–1195. [CrossRef] [PubMed]
12. El-Chami, M.F.; Bockstedt, L.; Longacre, C.; Higuera, L.; Stromberg, K.; Crossley, G.; Kowal, R.C.; Piccini, J.P. Leadless vs. transvenous single-chamber ventricular pacing in the Micra CED study: 2-year follow-up. *Eur. Heart J.* **2022**, *43*, 1207–1215. [CrossRef] [PubMed]
13. Burri, H. Leadless pacing: Is this the end of the road for transvenous pacemakers? *Eur. Heart J.* **2022**, *43*, 1216–1218. [CrossRef] [PubMed]
14. Fortescue, E.B.; Berul, C.I.; Cecchin, F.; Walsh, E.P.; Triedman, J.K.; Alexander, M.E. Patient, procedural, and hardware factors associated with pacemaker lead failures in pediatrics and congenital heart disease. *Heart Rhythm.* **2004**, *1*, 150–159. [CrossRef]
15. El-Chami, M.F.; Clementy, N.; Garweg, C.; Omar, R.; Duray, G.Z.; Gornick, C.C.; Leyva, F.; Sagi, V.; Piccini, J.P.; Soejima, K.; et al. Leadless Pacemaker Implantation in Hemodialysis Patients: Experience with the Micra Transcatheter Pacemaker. *JACC Clin. Electrophysiol.* **2019**, *5*, 162–170. [CrossRef] [PubMed]
16. Darlington, D.; Brown, P.; Carvalho, V.; Bourne, H.; Mayer, J.; Jones, N.; Walker, V.; Siddiqui, S.; Patwala, A.; Kwok, C.S. Efficacy and safety of leadless pacemaker: A systematic review, pooled analysis and meta-analysis. *Indian Pacing Electrophysiol. J.* **2022**, *22*, 77–86. [CrossRef] [PubMed]
17. Kirkfeldt, R.E.; Johansen, J.B.; Nohr, E.A.; Jørgensen, O.D.; Nielsen, J.C. Complications after cardiac implantable electronic device implantations: An analysis of a complete, nationwide cohort in Denmark. *Eur. Heart J.* **2014**, *35*, 1186–1194. [CrossRef]
18. Ngo, L.; Nour, D.; Denman, R.A.; Walters, T.E.; Haqqani, H.M.; Woodman, R.J.; Ranasinghe, I. Safety and Efficacy of Leadless Pacemakers: A Systematic Review and Meta-Analysis. *J. Am. Heart Assoc.* **2021**, *10*, e019212. [CrossRef]

19. Biffi, M.; Bertini, M.; Mazzotti, A.; Gardini, B.; Mantovani, V.; Ziacchi, M.; Valzania, C.; Martignani, C.; Diemberger, I.; Boriani, G. Long-term RV threshold behavior by automated measurements: Safety is the standpoint of pacemaker longevity! *J. Pacing Clin. Electrophysiol.* **2011**, *34*, 89–95. [CrossRef] [PubMed]
20. Kiani, S.; Wallace, K.; Stromberg, K.; Piccini, J.P.; Roberts, P.R.; El-Chami, M.F.; Soejima, K.; Garweg, C.; Fagan, D.H.; Lloyd, M.S. A Predictive Model for the Long-Term Electrical Performance of a Leadless Transcatheter Pacemaker. *JACC Clin. Electrophysiol.* **2021**, *7*, 502–512. [CrossRef] [PubMed]

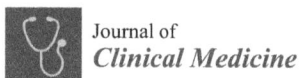
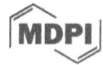

Article

Can the Norton Scale Score Be Used as an Adjunct Tool for Implantable Defibrillator Patient Selection? A Retrospective Single-Center Cohort Study

Shir Ben Asher Kestin [1,2,*,†], Ariel Israel [3,†], Eran Leshem [1,4], Anat Milman [1,4], Avi Sabbag [1,4], Ilan Goldengerg [5], Eyal Nof [1,4] and Roy Beinart [1,4,*]

1. Sackler Faculty of Medicine, Tel-Aviv University, Tel-Aviv 6997801, Israel
2. Department of Internal Medicine C, Meir Medical Center, Kfar-Saba 4428164, Israel
3. Leumit Research Institute, Leumit Health Services, Tel-Aviv 647378, Israel
4. Leviev Heart Center, Sheba Medical Center, Ramat Gan 5266202, Israel
5. Department of Medicine, School of Medicine and Dentistry, University of Rochester Medical Center, Rochester, NY 14642, USA
* Correspondence: shirba@gmail.com (S.B.A.K.); roy.beinart@sheba.health.gov.il (R.B.)
† These authors have contributed equally to this work and share first authorship.

Abstract: (1) Background: Implantable cardioverter defibrillators (ICDs) have become the standard of care in the prevention of sudden cardiac death, yet studies have shown that competing causes of death may limit ICD benefits. The Norton scale is a pressure ulcer risk score shown to have prognostic value in other fields. The purpose of this study was to assess the use of the Norton scale as an aid for ICD patient selection; (2) Methods: The study was comprised of consecutive patients who underwent defibrillator implantation at Sheba Medical Center between 2008 and 2016. A competing risk analysis was performed to assess the likelihood of death prior to device therapy; (3) Results: 695 patients were included. A total of 59 (8.5%) patients had low admission Norton scale score (ANSS) ($\leq$14), 81 (11.7%) had intermediate ANSS (15–17), and the remainder (79.8%) had high (18–20) ANSS. The cumulative probability of all-cause mortality within one year of ICD implantation in patients with low ANSS was 30%, compared with 20% and 7% among the intermediate- and high-ANSS groups, respectively. Moreover, the one-year mortality rate without ICD therapy in low-ANSS patients was over four-fold compared with that of high-ANSS patients (33% versus 7%, $p < 0.0001$); (4) Conclusions: The Norton scale could be a useful additional tool in predicting the life expectancy of ICD candidates, thereby improving patient selection.

Keywords: sudden cardiac death; implantable cardioverter device; Norton scale; pressure ulcer; patient selection

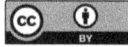

1. Introduction

Implantable cardioverter defibrillators (ICDs) have been previously shown to prevent sudden cardiac death in patients with reduced LV function [1,2] and in patients with a history of life-threatening arrhythmia or aborted sudden cardiac death [3]. ICD therapy is currently recommended in various indications by the ESC and AHA/ACC/HRS [4–6]. These guidelines, however, mandate that candidates for ICD implantation have a life expectancy of at least one year, with a reasonable functional status. In practice, it is difficult for clinicians to predict the survival of patients with heart failure [7–10]. Consequently, current patient selection for ICD implantation is challenging and remains sub-optimal, despite decades of experience. In fact, most patients who receive an ICD for primary prevention die of non-cardiac causes without utilizing life-saving shock therapy [10,11]. These findings suggest a need for improved methods for the prediction of life expectancy and better patient selection for ICD implantation.

Improper patient selection for ICD implantation imposes a considerable burden on health systems worldwide and exposes patients to unnecessary procedures and related complications [7,12].

Various stratification scales have been suggested as means to identify suitable candidates for defibrillator implantation [12–14]; however, none have been widely accepted in practice. Frailty has been shown to correlate with poor outcomes after ICD implantation [15], but the definition of frailty is non-uniform and it is assessed without consensus.

The Norton scale, originally purposed and used as a tool for pressure ulcer risk assessment, is routinely used by nursing staff in inpatient settings across the world, [16,17]. The scale evaluates five functional and clinical criteria (physical condition, mental condition, activity, mobility, and incontinence). For each criterion, the patient is given a score ranging from one to four, adding up to a total of five to twenty, with a lower score representing a higher risk (Table S1). The use of basic functional parameters contributes not only to its ease of use, but also to the applicability of the Norton scale to other fields, as it makes it indicative of the patients' basic general condition. Together with the fact that it is routinely calculated for patients on admission, the Norton scale appears to be an attractive tool for other stratification targets. Interestingly, the Norton scale has been suggested as a useful prognostic tool in many other disciplines, including cardiology [18,19]. The aim of this study was to evaluate the usefulness of the admission Norton scale score (ANSS) in identifying patients in whom ICD implantation would be futile, as their life expectancy would be less than one year.

2. Materials and Methods

Our study comprised a cohort of consecutive adult patients who underwent ICD or Cardiac Resynchronization Therapy with a Defibrillator (CRT-D) implantation or generator replacement at the Chaim Sheba Medical Center between January 2008 and June 2016. The routine device programming is detailed in Table S2. Following the approval of the institutional review and ethics board, patient data were retrospectively extracted from the electronic medical records. Patient records were maintained using a Chameleon® information system (Elad Healthcare Solutions).

The Norton score was computed at the time of admission by registered nurses using a dedicated computerized form as part of the mandatory admission protocol for all inpatients. Data collection was performed using Structured Query Language and custom Python/Pandas scripts accessing the Chameleon database. All patients aged 18 or above who underwent an ICD/CRT-D implantation or generator replacement during the study period were included.

The main study outcomes were all-cause mortality, appropriate defibrillation therapy, and death prior to defibrillation therapy. Data regarding defibrillator therapy were extracted from the devices during the regularly planned follow-up visits. Death events were queried from the Israel national population registry, with each patient identified by their unique national ID number. There were no patients lost to follow-up. The median follow-up time was 35 (IQR 22–49) months.

For descriptive statistics, we used the T-test to evaluate the statistical significance of differences in ordinal features distributed normally, the Kruskal–Wallis Rank Sum Test for non-normally distributed variables, and Fisher's exact test to compare categorical features. We used Kaplan–Meier's method to assess survival according to three predefined ANSS groups: low (≤ 14), intermediate (15–17), and high (18–20). Subgroup analyses were performed for patients with a reduced left ventricular ejection fraction (LVEF) ($\leq 35\%$) and for patients with high vs. low-risk clinical features (age ≥ 70 and/or creatinine ≥ 1.5 mg/dL) [20,21]. We further used COX proportional hazard models to calculate predictors of mortality in univariable models and multivariable models adjusted for age, gender, and comorbidities (CHF, Renal Disease, diabetes mellitus, and prior CVA); for multivariable models, we used backward stepwise selection to keep only significant predictors in the displayed models. Death without prior ICD therapy was assessed using a competing risk analysis among patients that did not receive shock therapy, i.e., patients who received shock were censored at the date of their first shock therapy and not further included in the population at risk. All statistical analyses were performed in R Statistical Language (R 3.5.1). $p < 0.05$ was considered significant.

3. Results

3.1. Cohort Population

Among the 695 study patients, the mean age was 66 ± 14 years, 85% were males, and the mean LVEF was $32 \pm 14\%$. Sixty-six percent underwent de-novo defibrillator implantations.

The cohort was divided into three pre-specified ANSS groups as routinely used in practice [22]: low (≤ 14), intermediate (15–17), and high (18–20) (Table S1). Due to the low number of patients with very low ANSS (<10), this group was included in the low (≤ 14) group. Most of the study population comprised the high-score group (79.8%), creating a leftward skew in the ANSS distribution, with a median of 19 (IQR 18–20) (Figure 1). A total of 59 patients (8.5%) had a low ANSS and 81 patients (11.7%) had an intermediate ANSS.

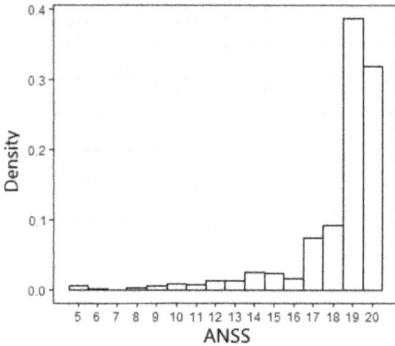

Figure 1. Distribution of admission Norton scale scores in the study population.

The baseline characteristics of the study population are shown in Table 1. Patients with lower ANSS were older and had significantly higher rates of heart failure, diabetes mellitus, and renal dysfunction, and a history of cerebrovascular accidents. Moreover, they had higher creatinine levels, as well as lower albumin and hemoglobin levels, representing their poor general condition. No major differences in medical treatment were noted.

Table 1. Baseline characteristics by admission Norton scale score.

Clinical Characteristics	Overall	ANSS $\leq$ 14	ANSS 15–17	ANSS 18–20	p Value
Study Population	$n = 695$	$n = 59$	$n = 81$	$n = 555$	
Age at procedure (years) $\pm$ SD	66 ± 14	70 ± 14	70 ± 12	65 ± 14	0.001
Female (%)	106 (15)	10 (17)	14 (17)	82 (15)	0.783
ANSS (median (IQR))	19 (18–20)	12 (10–14)	17 (16–17)	19 (19–20)	<0.001
High clinical risk * (%)	357 (51)	41 (70)	56 (69)	260 (47)	<0.001
De-novo ICD implantation (%)	461 (66)	42 (71)	52 (65)	367 (67)	0.734
Prior myocardial infarction (%)	262 (38)	19 (32)	33 (41)	210 (38)	0.546
Congestive heart failure (%)	345 (50)	37 (62)	49 (61)	259 (47)	0.008
Atrial fibrillation (%)	200 (29)	22 (37)	28 (35)	150 (27)	0.128
Prior CVA (%)	80 (12)	17 (29)	16 (20)	47 (9)	<0.001
Prior TIA (%)	19 (0.03)	1 (2)	1 (1)	17 (3)	0.560

Table 1. Cont.

Clinical Characteristics	Overall	ANSS ≤ 14	ANSS 15–17	ANSS 18–20	p Value
Study Population	n = 695	n = 59	n = 81	n = 555	
Dyslipidemia (%)	321 (46)	28 (48)	37 (46)	256 (46)	0.990
Currently on dialysis (%)	3 (0.004)	1 (2)	1 (1)	1 (0.2)	0.123
Hypertension (%)	358 (52)	31 (53)	47 (59)	280 (51)	0.430
Diabetes mellitus (%)	235 (34)	29 (49)	35 (44)	171 (31)	0.003
Smoker (%)	165 (24)	13 (22)	19 (24)	133 (24)	0.931
BMI (kg/m^2), ±SD	27 ± 5	27 ± 6	27 ± 5	27 ± 5	0.707
GFR MDRD (mL/min/1.73 m^2), ±SD	65 ± 32	66 ± 59	61 ± 26	66 ± 28	0.462
Serum creatinine (mg/dL), ±SD	1.3 ± 0.7	1.5 ± 1	1.4 ± 0.9	1.3 ± 0.6	0.024
Hemoglobin (g/dL), ±SD	13 ± 2	11 ± 2	12 ± 2	13 ± 2	<0.001
Serum albumin (g/dL), ±SD	4 ± 0.5	3 ± 0.6	4 ± 0.5	4 ± 0.4	<0.001
LV ejection fraction (%), ±SD	32 ± 14	33 ± 14	32 ± 14	32 ± 14	0.851
ACE inhibitors (%)	453 (65)	39 (66)	51 (63)	363 (65)	0.900
Aldosterone antagonists (%)	422 (61)	37 (63)	58 (72)	327 (59)	0.087
Beta-blockers (%)	185 (27)	17 (29)	17 (21)	151 (27)	0.459
Antiarrhythmics:					
Class IB (%)	27 (4)	3 (5)	4 (5)	20 (4)	0.746
Class IC (%)	23 (3)	2 (3)	3 (4)	18 (3)	0.976
Class III (%)	330 (47)	35 (59)	36 (44)	259 (47)	0.152
Salicylic acid (%)	13 (2)	0 (0)	1 (1)	12 (2)	0.458

* High clinical risk defined as age ≥ 70 years and/or baseline serum creatinine values ≥ 1.5 mg/dL. Values are the mean ± standard deviation, median (IQR), or n (%). ACE, angiotensin-converting enzyme; ANSS, admission Norton scale score; BMI, body mass index; CVA, cerebrovascular accident; GFR, glomerular filtration rate; ICD, implantable cardioverter defibrillator; LVEF, left-ventricular ejection fraction; MDRD, modification of diet in renal disease; TIA, transient ischemic attack.

3.2. All-Cause Mortality

Throughout the study period, 174 patients died; of those, 75 (43%) died within the first year following device implantation. In fact, the one-year mortality was significantly higher in patients with low ANSS (18 (30.5%)) compared with those with intermediate ANSS (16 (19.8%)) and with high ANSS (41 (7.4%)), ($p < 0.001$). The results were also consistent at two years after implantation: 27 (45.8%) patients from the low-ANSS group versus 22 (27.2%) and 74 (13.3%) patients from the intermediate- and high-ANSS groups, respectively ($p < 0.001$).

The Kaplan–Meier survival analysis demonstrates a statistically significant difference in the all-cause mortality at one year amongst the three Norton score groups, with the highest cumulative probability in the low-ANSS group (30%), compared with 20% and 7% among those in the intermediate- and high-ANSS groups, respectively. Likewise, at the two-year follow-up, the respective mortality probability rates were 46%, 27%, and 13% (log-rank p-value < 0.001 for the overall difference during follow-up; Figure 2).

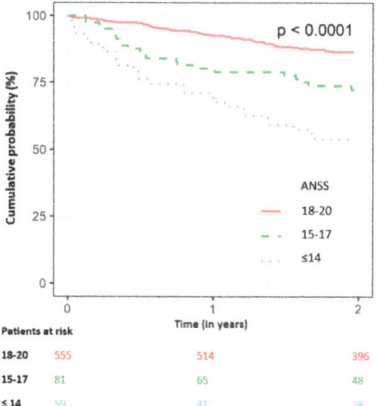

Figure 2. Kaplan–Meier Survival curve for all-cause mortality over time in the study population by admission Norton scale score. (Numbers reflect patients at risk. p value < 0.0001.) (ANSS, Admission Norton scale score).

3.3. Patients Not Receiving Appropriate ICD Therapy

We further assessed the risk of death for patients who did not receive appropriate ICD therapy at any time following implantation. At one year following implantation, 70 patients died without ICD therapy: 17 (28.8%) patients from the low-ANSS group versus 15 (18.5%) and 38 (6.8%) patients from the intermediate and high groups, respectively ($p < 0.001$). Similarly, at two years, 101 patients died without ICD therapy: 21 (35.6%) patients versus 19 (23.5%) and 61 (11%) patients, respectively ($p < 0.001$). Kaplan–Meier analysis showed a statistically significant association between mortality without ICD therapy and decreasing Norton score (Figure 3). The one-year probability of death without any ICD therapy following implantation among patients in the low-ANSS group was over four-fold higher compared with those with high ANSS (33% versus 7%). Similar findings were evident at two years following implantation (40% versus 12%) (log-rank p-value < 0.0001 for the overall difference during follow-up).

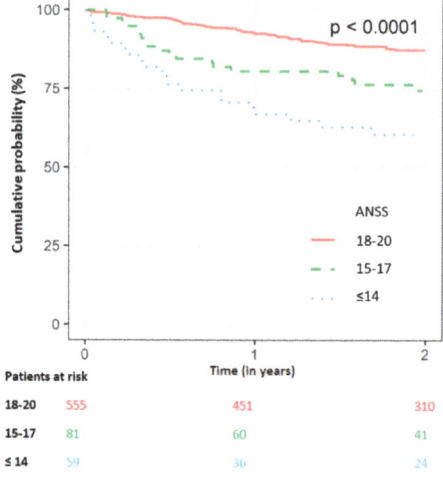

Figure 3. Kaplan–Meier survival curve for death without prior defibrillator therapy over time by admission Norton scale score (numbers reflect patients at risk. p value < 0.0001). (ANSS, Admission Norton scale score).

3.4. Association with Known Predictors of Poor Prognosis

Additionally, we evaluated the usefulness of ANSS in association with gender, age, and factors known to be associated with poor prognosis (congestive heart failure, diabetes mellitus, renal disease, and prior cerebrovascular accident) and performed a multivariate survival analysis using the Cox proportional hazards model adjusting for these variables. Our analysis demonstrates that, after adjusting to these significant factors, ANSS maintained its independent value. Patients in the low-ANSS group had a substantially higher risk of death from any cause compared with those in the high-ANSS group (HR: 2.39; 95% CI: 1.6–3.6; $p < 0.001$). Similarly, patients with intermediate ANSS had a higher risk of all-cause mortality compared with patients with high ANSS. (HR: 1.57; 95% CI: 1.03–2.39; $p = 0.036$) (Table 2). Likewise, the adjusted risk of death without prior ICD therapy was significantly higher in the low-ANSS group, and higher, albeit borderline significant, in the intermediate-ANSS group compared with the high-ANSS group (HR: 2.29; $p = 0.001$, and HR: 1.58; $p = 0.06$, respectively) (Table 3).

Table 2. COX proportional hazards univariable and multivariable models for all-cause mortality.

	Univariable Model			Multivariable Model		
	HR	95% CI	p	HR	95% CI	p
Age (year)	1.03	1.02–1.05	<0.001	1.02	1.00–1.03	0.018
Gender (Female)	0.73	0.46–1.16	0.179			
CHF	2.98	2.14–4.14	<0.001	2.15	1.52–3.04	<0.001
DM	1.66	1.23–2.25	<0.001			
Renal Disease	2.85	2.11–3.84	<0.001	1.89	1.37–2.61	<0.001
Prior CVA	1.54	1.02–2.32	0.040			
ANSS						
High (18–20) (reference)	1			1		—
Intermediate (15–17)	1.78	1.17–2.70	0.007	1.57	1.03–2.39	0.036
Low (≤14)	3.21	2.15–4.79	<0.001	2.39	1.59–3.60	<0.001

ANSS, admission Norton scale score; CHF, congestive heart failure; CVA, cerebrovascular accident; DM, diabetes mellitus.

Table 3. COX proportional hazards univariable and multivariable models for death without prior ICD therapy.

	Univariable Models			Multivariable Model		
	HR	95% CI	p	HR	95% CI	p
Age (year)	1.04	1.03–1.06	<0.001	1.02	1.01–1.04	0.010
Gender (Female)	0.68	0.40–1.17	0.163			
CHF	3.31	2.23–4.89	0.001	2.22	1.47–3.36	<0.001
DM	1.76	1.25–2.48	0.001			
Renal Disease	3.37	2.38–4.75	<0.001	2.12	1.46–3.07	<0.001
Prior CVA	1.69	1.08–2.65	0.023			
ANSS						
High (18–20) (reference)	1	—	—	1	—	—
Intermediate (15–17)	1.88	1.17–3.00	0.009	1.58	0.98–2.53	0.058
Low (≤14)	3.27	2.06–5.18	<0.001	2.29	1.44–3.77	0.001

ANSS, admission Norton scale score; CHF, congestive heart failure; CVA, cerebrovascular accident; DM, diabetes mellitus.

3.5. Subgroup Analysis

Additional analysis was performed for a subgroup of 448 patients with known LVEF $\leq 35\%$, representing the group of patients receiving ICD as indicated for cardiomyopathies and poor left ventricular function (Table S3). A Kaplan–Meyer analysis (Figures S1 and S2) yielded consistent results and showed higher mortality rates among patients with low ANSS (cumulative probabilities of all-cause mortality within one year for low versus high ANSS were 30% and 9% respectively, log rank $p < 0.0001$; for death without ICD therapy, the probabilities were 30% vs. 8%, respectively; log rank $p < 0.0001$).

We explored the utility of ANSS for risk stratification in patients with pre-defined high or low risk of mortality based on known clinical factors [20,21]. This sub-analysis showed that low ANSS remained a significant marker of increased all-cause mortality among patients with a high clinical risk of death (i.e., ≥ 70 years old and/or with baseline serum creatinine values ≥ 1.5 mg/dL), as well as in those with low clinical risk (i.e., <70 years old and with baseline serum creatinine values < 1.5 mg/dL) (Figure 4A,B). Notably, patients who had both a low ANSS and a high clinical risk experienced mortality rates at one year approaching 40% (Figure 4A). When applied to the subgroup of patients with LVEF $\leq 35\%$, our results remained consistent (Figure S3A,B).

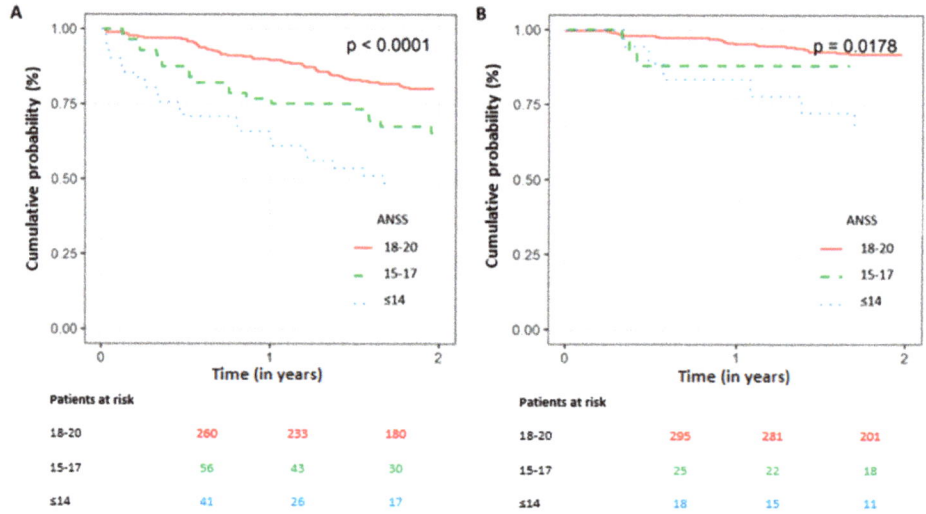

Figure 4. Kaplan–Meier survival curve for all-cause mortality over time in high vs. low clinical risk patients by admission Norton scale score. (**A**) High-clinical-risk patients: ≥ 70 years old and/or baseline serum creatinine values ≥ 1.5 mg/dL. *p* value < 0.0001. (**B**) Low-clinical-risk patients: <70 years old and baseline serum creatinine values < 1.5 mg/dL. *p* value = 0.0178. Numbers reflect patients at risk. ANSS, admission Norton scale score.

4. Discussion

Our findings show that patients with low ANSS were significantly more likely to die of any cause within one year of ICD implantation compared with high-ANSS patients. Moreover, they had a higher probability of dying without having received appropriate device therapy.

ICDs have become a fundamental part of the current guidelines for the prevention of sudden cardiac death in the setting of both primary and secondary prevention [4,5,23]. Nonetheless, the current guidelines require a life expectancy substantially over one year with reasonable functional status, a challenging decision for clinicians in the real-life setting [7,8]. Recent studies have shown that a high percentage of ICD recipients do not benefit from the device in real-life settings and, in fact, die of non-cardiac causes [10,11,24].

Improper patient selection imposes a considerable burden on health systems worldwide and exposes patients to unnecessary procedures and complications, such as infections and inappropriate device therapy [7,12,25], emphasizing the need for tools assisting in the identification of those who will not benefit from ICD therapy.

Previous studies have suggested various factors as possible markers for reduced survival following ICD implantation [12,20,21]. However, no single marker has been found to be as robust as LVEF [9]. In a recent observational study by Garcia et al. [26], regarding ICD for primary prevention, the combination of older age ($\geq$70), NYHA class $\geq$ III, and AF was associated with a 22.63% cumulative risk of mortality within one year of ICD implantation, but not as single markers. Similarly, different scoring systems and algorithms for the prediction of mortality in ICD-eligible patients have been suggested [13,14,27–30], but most are complex and none are currently used in practice. Our study suggests that the Norton scale, a simple and widely used pressure ulcer risk-assessment scale [16,17], could have high discriminative value for the prediction of non-cardiac mortality following ICD implantation. This scale has been previously shown to predict outcomes following trans-aortic valve implantation and myocardial infractions [18,19]. To our knowledge, it has not been used as a predictor of mortality in ICD recipients.

In this study, the cohort was divided into three prespecified ANSS groups (high risk, ANSS $\leq$ 14; medium risk, ANSS 15–17; and low risk, ANSS $\geq$ 18). We found that patients with ANSS $\leq$ 14 were significantly more likely to die of any cause for one year following ICD implantation and over four-fold more likely to die without having received appropriate device therapy compared with patients with ANSS $\geq$ 18. Our results remained significant at two years of follow-up and were validated by logistic regression models, proving the strength of the ANSS as a prognostic tool for ICD-implanted patients.

The endpoint of this study was all-cause mortality, and the cause of death was not specified, as mortality of any cause is the limiting factor for ICD implantation. Nevertheless, it would be of interest for further studies to focus on the relationship between the cause of death of these patients and ANSS. Of note, 75 patients (10.8% of the cohort) died within one year of device implantation, as compared with 6% for SCD-Heft [2] and 8% for MADIT-II [1]. Two recent studies regarding primary-prevention ICD had one-year mortality rates of 4.2% [26] and 4.8% [29]. Accurate rates of one-year mortality following ICD implantation are lacking, and great variation exists depending on the indication for implantation and etiology. Our population is greatly heterogeneous, as it is based on a single-center database and includes all implantations and replacements in the follow-up period. The fact that this study did not discriminate between de-novo implantations and device replacements is a limitation that requires further studies to address the value of the ANSS in these different patient populations. Still, a one-year life expectancy is required for all ICD recipients, and the requirements should ideally be re-evaluated before any device replacement, making this study relevant for the decision-making process.

Another limitation is that different ventricular fibrillation zone cut-offs were used according to the physicians' preferences and nominal values as determined by various vendors. This could possibly affect the rates of ICD therapies. Nevertheless, our primary finding of higher one-year mortality rates in ICD recipients with low ANSS should not be affected significantly by such nominal programming.

A recent systematic review by Chen et al., found that frailty in older patients, as assessed by various tools, is associated with a higher risk of mortality after ICD implantation for primary prevention [15], and various studies have shown that older age and renal failure are associated with poor outcomes following ICD implantation [20,21,31,32]. We, therefore, further explored the discriminative utility of the ANSS in these high-risk populations. Indeed, ANSS maintained its prognostic value in elderly patients and/or in patients with renal dysfunction. Hence, ANSS has independent prognostic value for survival, even in ICD recipients with high clinical risk, making it a potential supporting tool in the prediction of life expectancy and functional status for ICD candidates.

Our results demonstrate the possible value of ANSS in the assessment of ICD candidates having the potential to help and avoid futile implantation of defibrillators in patients with an ANSS of 14 or less. It showed that the one-year probability of death without ICD therapy in the low-ANSS group was over four-fold higher compared with that of the high-ANSS group, yet approximately two-thirds of patients did not die at one year without receiving ICD therapy. We suggest that combining the ANSS into the SCD-prevention decision-making process could provide support for clinicians in a real-life setting, but not as a stand-alone tool. Further prospective and randomized controlled studies are needed to validate these initial findings. If proven to have strong prognostic value in the appropriate populations in future studies, the use of the Norton scale could even be considered for incorporation into the guidelines for SCD prevention and assist in standardizing the currently ambiguous requirement for a life expectancy of at least one year.

5. Conclusions

Current guidelines for ICD implantation recommend a life expectancy of one year with reasonable functional status. The results of this study suggest that ANSS could be useful in the prediction of life expectancy in ICD candidates and might be used as a supportive tool, improving patient selection for ICD implantation.

Supplementary Materials: The following supporting information can be downloaded at: https://www.mdpi.com/article/10.3390/jcm12010214/s1, Figure S1: Kaplan–Meier Survival curve for all-cause mortality for patients with LVEF $\leq$ 35% over time by admission Norton scale score. Numbers reflect patients at risk. p value < 0.0001. ANSS = Admission Norton scale score; Figure S2: Kaplan–Meier Survival curve for death without prior defibrillator therapy in patients with LVEF $\leq$ 35% over time by admission Norton scale score. Numbers reflect patients at risk. p value < 0.0001. ANSS = Admission Norton scale score; Figure S3: Kaplan–Meier Survival curve for all-cause mortality over time in high vs. low clinical risk patients with LVEF $\leq$ 35%, by admission Norton scale score. Numbers reflect patients at risk. ANSS = Admission Norton scale score; Table S1: The Norton Pressure Sore Risk-Assessment Scale Scoring System; Table S2: Routine programming of implantable defibrillators in the Sheba medical center, Tel-Hashomer; Table S3: Baseline characteristics of patients with LVEF $\leq$ 35% by admission Norton scale score.

Author Contributions: Conceptualization: R.B. and I.G.; Methodology: R.B., I.G. and A.I.; Validation: A.S. and S.B.A.K.; Formal analysis: A.I.; Investigation: A.I. and S.B.A.K.; Resources: R.B. and A.S.; Data curation: A.I.; Writing—original draft preparation: S.B.A.K. and A.I.; Writing—review and editing: R.B., I.G., A.S., E.N., A.M. and E.L.; Visualization: S.B.A.K.; Supervision: R.B.; Project administration: S.B.A.K. All authors have read and agreed to the published version of the manuscript.

Funding: This research received no external funding.

Institutional Review Board Statement: The study was conducted in accordance with the Declaration of Helsinki and approved by the Institutional Review Board and Ethics Committee of Haim Sheba Medical Center. Approval number 9201000140 from 15 March 2010.

Informed Consent Statement: Patient consent was waived due to the retrospective nature of the study and the fact that the analyses used de-identified clinical data.

Data Availability Statement: Data are available upon request.

Acknowledgments: This work was partially performed in fulfillment of the M.D. thesis requirements for Shir Ben Asher Kestin at the Sackler Faculty of Medicine, Tel Aviv University.

Conflicts of Interest: The authors declare no conflict of interest.

References

1. Moss, A.J.; Zareba, W.; Hall, W.J.; Klein, H.; Wilber, D.J.; Cannom, D.S.; Daubert, J.P.; Higgins, S.L.; Brown, M.W.; Andrews, M.L. Prophylactic Implantation of a Defibrillator in Patients with Myocardial Infarction and Reduced Ejection Fraction. *N. Engl. J. Med.* **2002**, *346*, 877–883. [CrossRef] [PubMed]
2. Bardy, G.H.; Lee, K.L.; Mark, D.B.; Poole, J.E.; Packer, D.L.; Boineau, R.; Domanski, M.; Troutman, C.; Anderson, J.; Johnson, G.; et al. Amiodarone or an Implantable Cardioverter-Defibrillator for Congestive Heart Failure. *N. Engl. J. Med.* **2005**, *352*, 225–237. [CrossRef]
3. McAnulty, J.; Halperin, B.; Kron, J.; Larsen, G.; Raitt, M.; Swenson, R.; Florek, R.; Marchant, C.; Hamlin, M.; Heywood, G.; et al. A Comparison of Antiarrhythmic-Drug Therapy with Implantable Defibrillators in Patients Resuscitated from near-Fatal Ventricular Arrhythmias. *N. Engl. J. Med.* **1997**, *337*, 1576–1583. [CrossRef]
4. McDonagh, T.A.; Metra, M.; Adamo, M.; Gardner, R.S.; Baumbach, A.; Böhm, M.; Burri, H.; Butler, J.; Čelutkienė, J.; Chioncel, O.; et al. 2021 ESC Guidelines for the Diagnosis and Treatment of Acute and Chronic Heart Failure: Developed by the Task Force for the Diagnosis and Treatment of Acute and Chronic Heart Failure of the European Society of Cardiology (ESC) With the Special Contributio. *Eur. Heart J.* **2021**, *42*, 3599–3726. [CrossRef] [PubMed]
5. Lip, G.Y.H.; Heinzel, F.R.; Gaita, F.; Juanatey, J.R.G.; Le Heuzey, J.Y.; Potpara, T.; Svendsen, J.H.; Vos, M.A.; Anker, S.D.; Coats, A.J.; et al. European Heart Rhythm Association/Heart Failure Association Joint Consensus Document on Arrhythmias in Heart Failure, Endorsed by the Heart Rhythm Society and the Asia Pacific Heart Rhythm Society. *Eur. J. Heart Fail.* **2015**, *17*, 848–874. [CrossRef]
6. Zeppenfeld, K.; Tfelt-Hansen, J.; de Riva, M.; Winkel, B.G.; Behr, E.; Blom, N.; Charron, P.; Corrado, D.; Dagres, N.; de Chillou, C. 2022 ESC Guidelines for the Management of Patients with Ventricular Arrhythmias and the Prevention of Sudden Cardiac Death: Developed by the Task Force for the Management of Patients with Ventricular Arrhythmias and the Prevention of Sudden Cardiac Death. *Eur. Heart J.* **2022**, *43*, 3997–4126. [CrossRef]
7. Stevenson, L.W.; Desai, A.S. Selecting Patients for Discussion of the ICD as Primary Prevention for Sudden Death in Heart Failure. *J. Card. Fail.* **2006**, *12*, 407–412. [CrossRef]
8. Buxton, A.E.; Lee, K.L.; Hafley, G.E.; Pires, L.A.; Fisher, J.D.; Gold, M.R.; Josephson, M.E.; Lehmann, M.H.; Prystowsky, E.N. Limitations of Ejection Fraction for Prediction of Sudden Death Risk in Patients With Coronary Artery Disease. Lessons From the MUSTT Study. *J. Am. Coll. Cardiol.* **2007**, *50*, 1150–1157. [CrossRef]
9. Fishman, G.I.; Chugh, S.S.; Dimarco, J.P.; Albert, C.M.; Anderson, M.E.; Bonow, R.O.; Buxton, A.E.; Chen, P.S.; Estes, M.; Jouven, X.; et al. Sudden Cardiac Death Prediction and Prevention: Report from a National Heart, Lung, and Blood Institute and Heart Rhythm Society Workshop. *Circulation* **2010**, *122*, 2335–2348. [CrossRef]
10. Sabbag, A.; Suleiman, M.; Laish-Farkash, A.; Samania, N.; Kazatsker, M.; Goldenberg, I.; Glikson, M.; Beinart, R. Contemporary Rates of Appropriate Shock Therapy in Patients Who Receive Implantable Device Therapy in a Real-World Setting: From the Israeli ICD Registry. *Hear. Rhythm* **2015**, *12*, 2426–2433. [CrossRef]
11. Koller, M.T.; Schaer, B.; Wolbers, M.; Sticherling, C.; Bucher, H.C.; Osswald, S. Death Without Prior Appropriate Implantable Cardioverter-Defibrillator Therapy. *Circulation* **2008**, *117*, 1918–1926. [CrossRef]
12. Disertori, M.; Quintarelli, S.; Mazzola, S.; Favalli, V.; Narula, N.; Arbustini, E. The Need to Modify Patient Selection to Improve the Benefits of Implantable Cardioverter-Defibrillator for Primary Prevention of Sudden Death in Non-Ischaemic Dilated Cardiomyopathy. *Europace* **2013**, *15*, 1693–1701. [CrossRef] [PubMed]
13. Goldenberg, I.; Vyas, A.K.; Hall, W.J.; Moss, A.J.; Wang, H.; He, H.; Zareba, W.; McNitt, S.; Andrews, M.L. Risk Stratification for Primary Implantation of a Cardioverter-Defibrillator in Patients With Ischemic Left Ventricular Dysfunction. *J. Am. Coll. Cardiol.* **2008**, *51*, 288–296. [CrossRef] [PubMed]
14. Kaura, A.; Sunderland, N.; Kamdar, R.; Petzer, E.; McDonagh, T.; Murgatroyd, F.; Dhillon, P.; Scott, P. Identifying Patients with Less Potential to Benefit from Implantable Cardioverter-Defibrillator Therapy: Comparison of the Performance of Four Risk Scoring Systems. *J. Interv. Card. Electrophysiol.* **2017**, *49*, 181–189. [CrossRef] [PubMed]
15. Chen, M.Y.; Orkaby, A.R.; Rosenberg, M.A.; Driver, J.A. Frailty, Implantable Cardioverter Defibrillators, and Mortality: A Systematic Review. *J. Gen. Intern. Med.* **2019**, *34*, 2224–2231. [CrossRef] [PubMed]
16. Šateková, L.; Žiaková, K.; Zeleníková, R. Predictive Validity of the Braden Scale, Norton Scale, and Waterlow Scale in the Czech Republic. *Int. J. Nurs. Pract.* **2017**, *23*, e12499. [CrossRef]
17. Norton, D.; Exton-Smith, A.N.; McLaren, R. An Investigation of Geriatric Nursing Problems in Hospital. *Br. J. Psychiatry* **1963**, *109*, 152–153. [CrossRef]
18. Silber, H.; Shiyovich, A.; Gilutz, H.; Ziedenberg, H.; Abu Tailakh, M.; Plakht, Y. Decreased Norton's Functional Score Is an Independent Long-Term Prognostic Marker in Hospital Survivors of Acute Myocardial Infarction. Soroka Acute Myocardial Infarction II (SAMI-II) Project. *Int. J. Cardiol.* **2017**, *228*, 694–699. [CrossRef]
19. Rabinovitz, E.; Finkelstein, A.; Ben Assa, E.; Steinvil, A.; Konigstein, M.; Shacham, Y.; Yankelson, L.; Banai, S.; Justo, D.; Leshem-Rubinow, E. Norton Scale for Predicting Prognosis in Elderly Patients Undergoing Trans-Catheter Aortic Valve Implantation: A Historical Prospective Study. *J. Cardiol.* **2016**, *67*, 519–525. [CrossRef]
20. Goldenberg, I.; Moss, A.J.; McNitt, S.; Zareba, W.; Andrews, M.L.; Hall, W.J.; Greenberg, H.; Case, R.B. Relations Among Renal Function, Risk of Sudden Cardiac Death, and Benefit of the Implanted Cardiac Defibrillator in Patients With Ischemic Left Ventricular Dysfunction. *Am. J. Cardiol.* **2006**, *98*, 485–490. [CrossRef]

21. Cuculich, P.S.; Sánchez, J.M.; Kerzner, R.; Greenberg, S.L.; Sengupta, J.; Chen, J.; Faddis, M.N.; Gleva, M.J.; Smith, T.W.; Lindsay, B.D. Poor Prognosis for Patients with Chronic Kidney Disease despite ICD Therapy for the Primary Prevention of Sudden Death. *PACE—Pacing Clin. Electrophysiol.* **2007**, *30*, 207–213. [CrossRef] [PubMed]
22. Reilly, E.F.; Karakousis, G.C.; Schrag, S.P.; Stawicki, S. Pressure Ulcers in the Intensive Care Unit: The "forgotten" Enemy. *OPUS 12 Sci.* **2007**, *1*, 17–30.
23. Al-Khatib, S.M.; Stevenson, W.G.; Ackerman, M.J.; Bryant, W.J.; Callans, D.J.; Curtis, A.B.; Deal, B.J.; Dickfeld, T.; Field, M.E.; Fonarow, G.C.; et al. 2017 AHA/ACC/HRS Guideline for Management of Patients With Ventricular Arrhythmias and the Prevention of Sudden Cardiac Death. *Circulation* **2018**, *138*, e272–e391. [CrossRef]
24. Køber, L.; Thune, J.J.; Nielsen, J.C.; Haarbo, J.; Videbæk, L.; Korup, E.; Jensen, G.; Hildebrandt, P.; Steffensen, F.H.; Bruun, N.E.; et al. Defibrillator Implantation in Patients with Nonischemic Systolic Heart Failure. *N. Engl. J. Med.* **2016**, *375*, 1221–1230. [CrossRef] [PubMed]
25. Hajduk, A.M.; Gurwitz, J.H.; Tabada, G.; Masoudi, F.A.; Magid, D.J.; Greenlee, R.T.; Sung, S.H.; Cassidy-Bushrow, A.E.; Liu, T.I.; Reynolds, K.; et al. Influence of Multimorbidity on Burden and Appropriateness of Implantable Cardioverter-Defibrillator Therapies. *J. Am. Geriatr. Soc.* **2019**, *67*, 1370–1378. [CrossRef] [PubMed]
26. Garcia, R.; Boveda, S.; Defaye, P.; Sadoul, N.; Narayanan, K.; Perier, M.-C.; Klug, D.; Fauchier, L.; Leclercq, C.; Babuty, D.; et al. Early Mortality after Implantable Cardioverter Defibrillator: Incidence and Associated Factors. *Int. J. Cardiol.* **2020**, *301*, 114–118. [CrossRef] [PubMed]
27. Parkash, R.; Stevenson, W.G.; Epstein, L.M.; Maisel, W.H. Predicting Early Mortality after Implantable Defibrillator Implantation: A Clinical Risk Score for Optimal Patient Selection. *Am. Heart J.* **2006**, *151*, 397–403. [CrossRef]
28. Kramer, D.B.; Friedman, P.A.; Kallinen, L.M.; Morrison, T.B.; Crusan, D.J.; Hodge, D.O.; Reynolds, M.R.; Hauser, R.G. Development and Validation of a Risk Score to Predict Early Mortality in Recipients of Implantable Cardioverter-Defibrillators. *Hear. Rhythm* **2012**, *9*, 42–46. [CrossRef]
29. Kraaier, K.; Scholten, M.F.; Tijssen, J.G.P.; Theuns, D.A.M.J.; Jordaens, L.J.L.M.; Wilde, A.A.M.; van Dessel, P.F.H.M. Early Mortality in Prophylactic Implantable Cardioverter-Defibrillator Recipients: Development and Validation of a Clinical Risk Score. *EP Eur.* **2014**, *16*, 40–46. [CrossRef]
30. Younis, A.; Goldberger, J.J.; Kutyifa, V.; Zareba, W.; Polonsky, B.; Klein, H.; Aktas, M.K.; Huang, D.; Daubert, J.; Estes, M.; et al. Predicted Benefit of an Implantable Cardioverter-Defibrillator: The MADIT-ICD Benefit Score. *Eur. Heart J.* **2021**, *42*, 1676–1684. [CrossRef]
31. Bansal, N.; Szpiro, A.; Reynolds, K.; Smith, D.H.; Magid, D.J.; Gurwitz, J.H.; Masoudi, F.; Greenlee, R.T.; Tabada, G.H.; Sung, S.H.; et al. Long-Term Outcomes Associated With Implantable Cardioverter Defibrillator in Adults With Chronic Kidney Disease. *JAMA Intern. Med.* **2018**, *178*, 390–398. [CrossRef] [PubMed]
32. Jukema, J.W.; Timal, R.J.; Rotmans, J.I.; Hensen, L.C.R.; Buiten, M.S.; de Bie, M.K.; Putter, H.; Zwinderman, A.H.; van Erven, L.; Straaten, M.J.K.; et al. Prophylactic Use of Implantable Cardioverter-Defibrillators in the Prevention of Sudden Cardiac Death in Dialysis Patients. *Circulation* **2019**, *139*, 2628–2638. [CrossRef] [PubMed]

Disclaimer/Publisher's Note: The statements, opinions and data contained in all publications are solely those of the individual author(s) and contributor(s) and not of MDPI and/or the editor(s). MDPI and/or the editor(s) disclaim responsibility for any injury to people or property resulting from any ideas, methods, instructions or products referred to in the content.

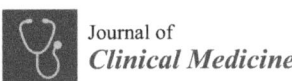

Article

Left Ventricular "Longitudinal Rotation" and Conduction Abnormalities—A New Outlook on Dyssynchrony

Ibrahim Marai [1,2,*], Rabea Haddad [1,2], Nizar Andria [1,2], Wadi Kinany [1,2], Yevgeni Hazanov [1,2], Bruce M. Kleinberg [1,2], Edo Birati [1,2] and Shemy Carasso [1,2]

[1] The Lydia and Carol Kittner, Lea and Benjamin Davidai Division of Cardiovascular Medicine and Surgery, Baruch Padeh Poriya Medical Center, Poriya 1528001, Israel
[2] The Azrieli Faculty of Medicine, Bar Ilan University, Zefat 1311502, Israel
* Correspondence: imarai@poria.health.gov.il

Abstract: Background: The complete left bundle branch block (CLBBB) results in ventricular dyssynchrony and a reduction in systolic and diastolic efficiency. We noticed a distinct clockwise rotation of the left ventricle (LV) in patients with CLBBB ("longitudinal rotation"). Aim: The aim of this study was to quantify the "longitudinal rotation" of the LV in patients with CLBBB in comparison to patients with normal conduction or complete right bundle branch block (CRBBB). Methods: Sixty consecutive patients with normal QRS, CRBBB, or CLBBB were included. Stored raw data DICOM 2D apical-4 chambers view images cine clips were analyzed using EchoPac plugin version 203 (GE Vingmed Ultrasound AS, Horten, Norway). In EchoPac-Q-Analysis, 2D strain application was selected. Instead of apical view algorithms, the SAX-MV (short axis—mitral valve level) algorithm was selected for analysis. A closed loop endocardial contour was drawn to initiate the analysis. The "posterior" segment (representing the mitral valve) was excluded before finalizing the analysis. Longitudinal rotation direction, peak angle, and time-to-peak rotation were recorded. Results: All patients with CLBBB ($n = 21$) had clockwise longitudinal rotation with mean four chamber peak rotation angle of $-3.9 \pm 2.4°$. This rotation is significantly larger than in patients with normal QRS ($-1.4 \pm 3°$, $p = 0.005$) and CRBBB ($0.1 \pm 2.2°$, $p = 0.00001$). Clockwise rotation was found to be correlated to QRS duration in patients with the non-RBBB pattern. The angle of rotation was not associated with a lower ejection fraction or the presence of regional wall abnormalities. Conclusions: Significant clockwise longitudinal rotation was found in CLBBB patients compared to normal QRS or CRBBB patients using speckle-tracking echocardiography.

Keywords: CLBBB; clockwise; longitudinal; rotation

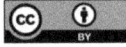

1. Introduction

Left ventricular contraction efficiency depends in part on synchronous activation of the myocardium. Synchronous activation depends on atrioventricular (AV) synchrony, inter-ventricular (left and right ventricle) synchrony, and intra-ventricular synchrony (within left ventricle). AV synchrony depends on AV conduction, and inter-ventricular synchrony on having intact, fully functioning right and left bundle branches. Intra-ventricular synchrony needs an intact, fully functional left bundle branch and associated subdivisions.

When the conduction system is intact, there is a simultaneous contraction of the myocardium, resulting in efficient systolic and diastolic function. In contrast, conduction delay as in complete left bundle branch block (CLBBB) results in sequential contraction and ventricular dyssynchrony that reduces systolic and diastolic efficiency [1]. Many methods of assessment of this dyssynchrony have been previously suggested at the beginning of the era of cardiac resynchronization therapy (CRT) to pre-assess its presence and extent and optimize results after device implantation [2]. These included use of multiple 2D-Doppler echocardiographic methodologies as m-mode [3], tissue Doppler imaging [4–7], tissue strain timing [8,9], and tissue strain patterns [10].

Novel strain-imaging techniques using speckle-tracking echocardiography can provide information about regional myocardial mechanics, including not only the timing of myocardial contraction but also patterns of mechanical dysfunction [10]. However, in daily practice when viewing the left ventricle in the apical four chamber view, we noticed a distinct clockwise longitudinal rotation of the left ventricle in patients with CLBBB not addressed by the traditional longitudinal, circumferential, or radial strains that are assessed by speckle-tracking echocardiography. This unique rotation was previously reported by Popovic' et al. in patients with dilated cardiomyopathy [11].

The aim of this study was to quantify this "longitudinal rotation" of the left ventricle in patients with CLBBB in comparison to patients with normal conduction or complete right bundle branch block (CRBBB) using speckle-tracking echocardiography in an unorthodox way with application of circumferential assessment strain-imaging tools on longitudinal apical long axis views.

2. Methods

2.1. Patient Selection

This retrospective study included three groups of patients based on the QRS pattern: patients with normal QRS, patients with CLBBB, and patients with CRBBB. We selected consecutive patients for each pattern who had comprehensive echocardiography at the Poriya Medical Center in northern Israel: 19 patients with normal QRS duration and normal ejection fraction, 20 patients with CRBBB and preserved ejection fraction, and 21 patients with CLBBB. Clinical and echocardiographic data were extracted from the institute's database. The indications for echocardiographic studies were dyspnea and chest pain. QRS pattern and width were determined from ECG tracings that were recorded on the same day of the echocardiographic studies. This study was approved by the local ethical institutional committee.

2.2. Echocardiography

Echocardiography (2D-Doppler) was done according to the ASE/EACAVI guidelines [12] on various ultrasound machines (GE Vivid i, E9, E95). Cine clips were stored in full frame rate and not compressed to enable subsequent off-line analysis Ejection fraction, regional wall abnormality (qualitatively analyzed), systolic and diastolic dimensions, and valvular abnormalities were recorded.

2.3. Longitudinal Rotation Quantification

The longitudinal strain algorithm is designed to detect myocardial displacement towards the apex. To measure longitudinal rotation, a circumferential strain algorithm is used to assess radial motion relative to a centroid of the ventricle. This method allows one to calculate the direction and extent (peak angle) of the longitudinal rotation [11].

Stored raw data DICOM 2D apical-4 chamber view cine image clips were analyzed using EchoPac plugin version 203 (GE Vingmed Ultrasound AS, Horten, Norway). All analyses were performed offline by a single experienced cardiologist (S.C) specialized in 2D strain imaging. In EchoPac-Q-Analysis, 2D strain application was selected. Instead of using the apical view algorithm for longitudinal strain assessment, the SAX-MV (short axis—mitral valve level) algorithm, used for circumferential strain assessment, was selected for analysis and assessment of "longitudinal rotation". A closed-loop endocardial contour was drawn to initiate the analysis. After assuring good tracking, the "posterior" segment (representing the mitral valve annulus) was excluded before finalizing the analysis. Longitudinal rotation direction, peak angle, and time-to-peak rotation were recorded.

2.4. Statistical Analysis

Categorical variables were expressed as percentages and continuous variables as means ± standard deviations. Pattern characteristics were compared using ANOVA with the Tukey–Kramer post-hoc analysis. Correlation between QRS duration and longitudinal rotation angles were performed using a two-side regression analysis. Chi-square analysis was used for categorical variables. Sensitivity and specificity of longitudinal rotation analysis for the identification of CLBBB was done using ROC (receiver operating characteristic) curve analysis. Statistical significance was defined as a p value < 0.05.

Statistical analyses were performed using the MedCalc Statistical Software version 15.6.1 (MedCalc Software bvba, Ostend, Belgium).

3. Results

3.1. Clinical and Echocardiographic Data

The clinical and echocardiographic data are presented in Table 1. Sixty patients were included in the study: 19 patients with a normal QRS pattern, 21 patients with a CLBBB pattern, and 20 patients with a CRBBB pattern. The mean age of the CLBBB patients (67 ± 12 years) and the CRBBB patients (71 ± 13 years) was significantly higher than the normal QRS patients (61 ± 14 years). Female gender constituted 31.6% of the normal QRS patients, 33.3% of the CLBBB patients, and 25% of the CRBBB patients without significant differences between groups. The QRS duration was shorter among the normal QRS patients with a duration of 95 ± 8 ms, compared to the CLBBB patients (159 ± 15 ms, p = 0.00001) and the CRBBB patients (141 ± 11 ms, p = 0.0001). On the other hand, the QRS duration of the CRBBB patients was shorter than the CLBBB patients (p = 0.0001). The ejection fraction was higher among the normal QRS patients (62 ± 6%) compared to the CRBBB patients (55 ± 14%, p = 0.038) and the CLBBB patients (45 ± 17%, p = 0.0001). The ejection fraction among the CRBBB patients was higher than the ejection fraction among the CLBBB patients (p = 0.043). The left ventricular end diastolic diameter was larger among the CLBBB patients (61 ± 12 mm) compared to the normal QRS patients (53 ± 4 mm) and the CRBBB patients (54 ± 10 mm). The left ventricular end systolic diameter was also larger among the CLBBB patients (47 ± 14 mm) compared to the normal QRS patients (34 ± 5 mm) and the CRBBB patients (38 ± 12 mm). Regional wall motion abnormalities were more common among the CLBBB patients (38.1%) compared to the normal QRS patients (10.5%, p = 0.044) and tended to be more common among the CRBBB patients (35%) compared to the normal QRS patients (p = 0.07). Congestive heart failure was more frequent among the CLBBB patients (66.7%) compared to the normal QRS patients (5.3%, 0.00006) or the CRBBB patients (30%, p = 0.02). On the other hand, congestive heart failure was more common among the CRBBB patients compared to the normal QRS patients (p = 0.044).

3.2. Longitudinal Rotation

The SAX-MV (short axis—mitral valve level) algorithm used for circumferential strain assessment was easily applied for assessment of "longitudinal rotation" in all participants. Longitudinal rotation angles differed according to conduction patterns (normal QRS, CRBBB, or CLBBB), as demonstrated in Figure 1. In the CLBBB pattern, there was definite and extensive longitudinal clockwise rotation. All patients with CLBBB (n = 21) had clockwise rotation with mean four chamber peak rotation angle of $-3.9 \pm 2.4°$ degrees (Figure 2).

In a CRBBB pattern, there was definite and extensive longitudinal counterclockwise rotation. However, this rotation pattern was variable among patients with CRBBB. We found 65% of CRBBB patients had counterclockwise rotation, while 35% had clockwise rotation. CRBBB patients had a significantly lower rate of clockwise rotation compared to the CLBBB patients. Overall, patients with CRBBB had minimal mean rotation (0.1 ± 2.2°), which was significantly less than patients with CLBBB (p = 0.00001). In patients with a normal QRS pattern (no conduction delay), minimal clockwise rotation was observed. Normal QRS patients had an average rotation of $-1.4 \pm 3°$, which was significantly less than the CLBBB patients (p = 0.005) but not significantly different from the CRBBB patients (p = 0.093) (Table 1). Clockwise rotation was found among 58% of the normal QRS patients which was not significantly different than among the CRBBB patients (35%, p = 0.15) but significantly lower than the CLBBB patients.

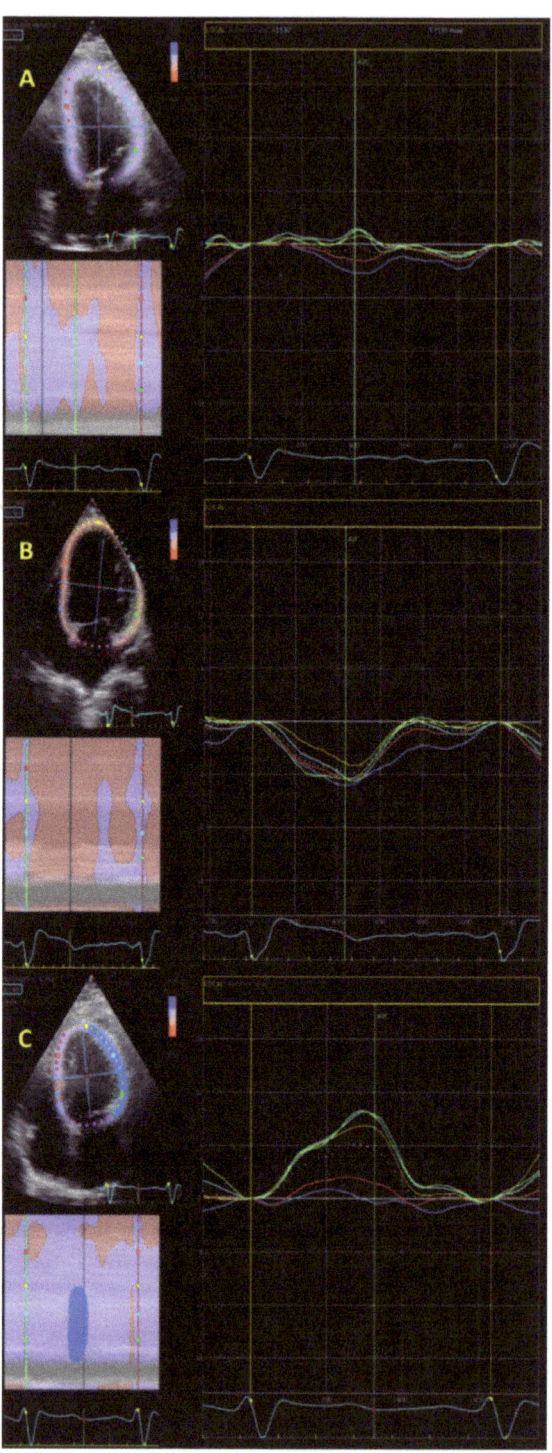

Figure 1. Examples of longitudinal rotation direction and extent in the various patterns analyzed using circumferential rotation algorithm on longitudinal images. Note the "posterior" or annular

segment (in pink color) was excluded from analysis. The dotted lines represent the average rotation curve. (**A**)—Normal QRS duration, no conduction delay. Note the minimal clockwise rotation. (**B**)—CLBBB pattern. Definite and extensive longitudinal clockwise rotation. (**C**)—CRBBB pattern. Definite and extensive longitudinal counterclockwise rotation. This rotation pattern was variable among patients with CRBBB.

Table 1. Clinical and echocardiographic data.

	Normal (n = 19)	LBBB (n = 21)	p Value (LBBB vs. Normal)	RBBB (n = 20)	p Value (RBBB vs. Normal)	p Value (LBBB vs. RBBB)
Age	61 ± 14	67 ± 12	0.0497	71 ± 13	0.008	0.16
Female gender n, %	6 (31.6)	7 (33.3)	0.9	5 (25)	0.65	0.56
QRS duration (ms)	95 ± 8	159 ± 15	0.00001	141 ± 11	0.00001	0.00001
Heart rate (min^{-1})	70 ± 12	78 ± 21	0.17	75 ± 13	0.24	0.56
Ejection fraction (%)	62 ± 6	45 ± 17	0.0001	55 ± 14	0.038	0.043
LVEDD (mm)	53 ± 4	61 ± 12	0.004	54 ± 10	0.2	0.04
LVESD (mm)	34 ± 5	47 ± 14	0.0002	38 ± 12	0.06	0.02
Severe valvular disease n, %	1 (5.3)	5 (23.8)	0.1	6 (30)	0.1	0.9
Regional WMA n, %	2 (10.5)	8 (38.1)	0.044	7 (35)	0.07	0.8
CHF n, %	1 (5.3)	14 (66.7)	0.00006	6 (30)	0.044	0.02
Clockwise rotation n, %	11 (58)	21 (100)	<0.005	7 (35)	0.15	<0.0005
Longitudinal rotation angle (°)	−1.4 ± 3	−3.9 ± 2.4	0.005	0.1 ± 2.2	0.093	0.00001
Time to peak rotation (ms)	395 ± 98	339 ± 135	0.1447	367 ± 89	0.356	0.437

WMA—wall motion abnormality, CHF—congestive heart failure, LBBB—left bundle branch block, RBBB—right bundle branch block, LVEDD—left ventricular end diastolic diameter, LVESD-left ventricular end systolic diameter.

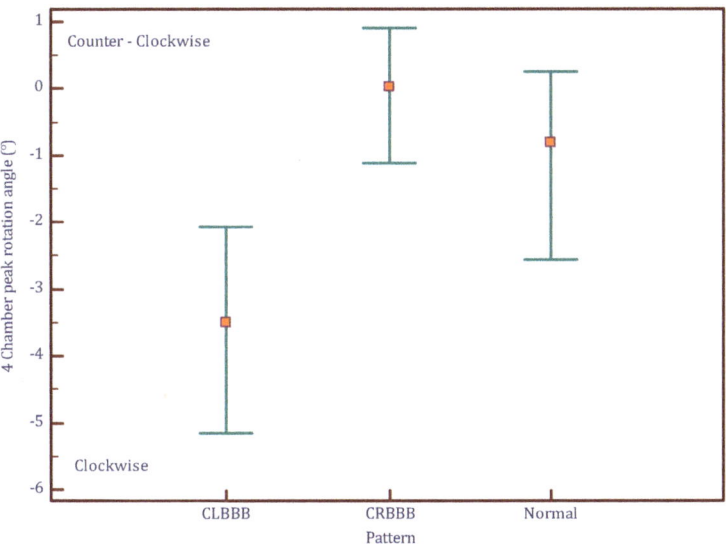

Figure 2. Comparison of longitudinal rotation angle according to conduction pattern. Negative angles are for clockwise rotation, and positive angles are for counterclockwise rotation.

Using regression analysis, clockwise rotation was found to be correlated to QRS duration in patients with a non-RBBB pattern (LBBB pattern and normal QRS pattern) (Figure 3). As shown in Figure 3, a longer QRS duration resulted in more clockwise rotation (more negative peak rotation angle). Time-to-peak rotation was not different among the groups: 395 ± 98 ms in normal QRS patients, 339 ± 135 ms in CLBBB patients, and 367 ± 89 ms in CRBBB patients.

Identification of a CLBBB pattern using longitudinal rotation was found to be 95% sensitive and 62% specific for a longitudinal rotation angle smaller or equal to −0.9° (larger negative means more clockwise longitudinal rotation) with an AUC of 0.85 and a p-value of <0.001, as seen in ROC curve analysis in Figure 4.

Importantly, the angle of longitudinal rotation was not associated with low ejection fraction or the presence of regional wall abnormality or the echocardiography machine used.

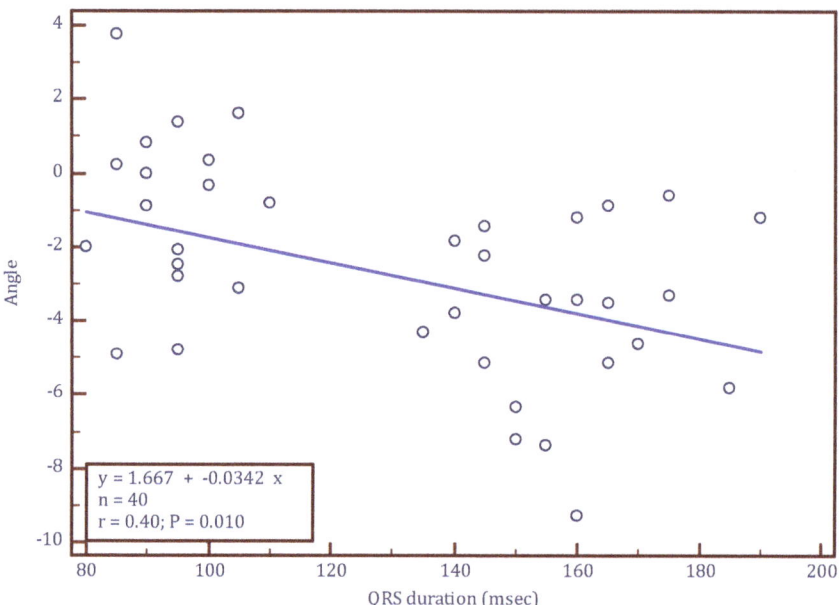

Figure 3. Regression analysis of QRS duration (ms) and longitudinal rotation angle, excluding the CRBBB group.

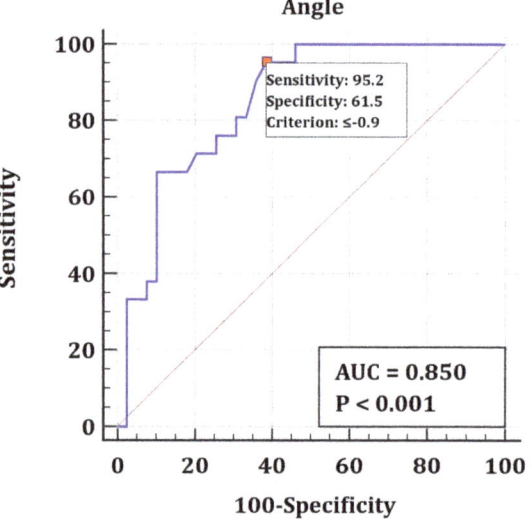

Figure 4. ROC analysis for identification of CLBBB pattern according to rotation angle.

4. Discussion

4.1. Main Findings

The main findings of this study were: (i) definite and extensive clockwise longitudinal rotation in CLBBB patients, (ii) minimal clockwise or counterclockwise rotation in normal or CRBBB patients, (iii) the angle of clockwise longitudinal rotation correlated with QRS duration in patients with non-RBBB pattern, (iv) the angle of rotation was not associated with low ejection fraction or the presence of regional wall abnormality or the echocardiography machine used.

4.2. Longitudinal Rotation

For quantification of longitudinal rotation, we used 2D speckle-tracking echocardiography that has been used for evaluating myocardial mechanics in the last decade as did Popovic' et al. [11,13]. This method allows for the measurement of left ventricular strain and volume changes throughout the cardiac cycle. Longitudinal, circumferential, and radial strain can be measured easily using dedicated software and appropriate views. Standard strain software assesses rotation only in short axis. Thus, to assess and quantify longitudinal left ventricular rotation and its relation to conduction abnormalities, we applied the short axis strain tool used for circumferential strain on the apical four chamber view used for longitudinal strain. In contrast to Popovic' et al., we used more than one echocardiography machine, and we excluded the "posterior" segment (representing the mitral valve) before finalizing the analysis.

Our findings confirmed the direction of longitudinal rotation in CLBBB patients was consistent with that expected from daily practice, and its magnitude correlated with the QRS duration (a wider QRS duration in CLBBB patients correlated with more longitudinal clockwise rotation). This finding may explain the mechanical consequences of CLBBB on myocardial function and add to our general base of knowledge on the matter. As it is well known, CLBBB can cause left ventricular dyssynchrony. This dyssynchrony is heterogeneous and depends on the width of the QRS interval and the degree of left ventricular function. Rao et al. [14] reported 72% of heart failure patients with LBBB have documented dyssynchrony on tissue Doppler imaging, which has a heterogeneous regional distribution. Dyssynchrony may be seen in LBBB and normal hearts, but it is does not involve the lateral wall [14]. Contraction patterns in classical CLBBB based on 2D speckle-tracking echocardiographic longitudinal strain analysis (when the septal peak shortening occurred within the initial 70% of the ejection phase, and the lateral wall was initially stretched and had peak shortening after aortic valve closure) were previously reported [15]. This classical contraction pattern has been associated with improved echocardiographic function and survival without the need for heart transplantation or left ventricular assist device implantation in CRT recipients, independent of QRS duration and ischemic etiology [15,16]. Furthermore, a classical CLBBB contraction pattern on longitudinal strain analysis was associated with a better outcome in CRT recipients evaluated by strain software [17]. Recently, Calle et al. proposed a classification of LBBB induced cardiac remodeling based on longitudinal strain patterns [18]. The proposed classification suggests a pathophysiological continuum of LBBB-induced left ventricular remodeling and may be valuable to assess the contribution of LBBB to the degree of left ventricular remodeling and dysfunction. All the mentioned methods rely on timing of activation for evaluation of dyssynchrony and response to CRT and were unable to fully describe mechanical dyssynchrony, the actual target of CRT [10]. Carasso et al. reported left ventricular mechanical strain patterns, rather than just showing the timing of activation, were also found to be highly predictive of the response to CRT [10]. Erikson et al. reported unique flow-specific measures of mechanical dyssynchrony in heart failure patients with LBBB that may serve as an additional tool for considering the risks imposed by conduction abnormalities in heart failure patients and prove to be useful in predicting responses to CRT [19]. However, the last method is based on cardiac MRI, which is not widely used in clinical practice.

A substantial proportion of patients receiving CRT do not improve their functional or echocardiographic status [20,21], regardless of the pre-implantation assessment methods or the post-implantation assessment of resynchronization used. Our method may help in classification of LBBB-induced cardiac remodeling based on longitudinal rotation patterns. This study demonstrated high sensitivity for identification of CLBBB patterns using longitudinal rotation. It may help in predicting the response to CRT by easy identification and quantification of futile myocardial work of longitudinal rotation. Furthermore, this method may help in optimizing CRT after implantation by iterating changes in V-V intervals to minimize the clockwise longitudinal rotation. Clinical studies are needed to validate this method and its additive value over the available clinical, echocardiographic, or device-based optimization techniques [22].

Strain measures myocardial deformation in three dimensions; myocardial shortening from base to apex by longitudinal strain, systolic shortening of the short axis of the ventricle by circumferential strain, and myocardial thickening from endocardium to epicardium by radial strain [23]. One study assessed the usefulness of each type of strain (radial, circumferential, and longitudinal strain) for left ventricular dyssynchrony assessment and its predictive value for a positive response after cardiac CRT. In this study, speckle-tracking radial strain analysis constituted the best method to identify potential responders to CRT [24]. Other studies found combined patterns of longitudinal and radial dyssynchrony could be predictive of left ventricular functional response after CRT [8]. Helm et al. reported dyssynchrony assessed by longitudinal motion was less sensitive to dyssynchrony and followed different time courses than those assessments that utilized circumferential motion [25]. Wang et al. reported the LBBB-contraction pattern identified from radial-strain analysis in the mid-ventricular short-axis view predicted reverse remodeling and outcome following CRT, similar to the longitudinal-strain analysis [26]. Delgado-Montero et al. reported baseline global circumferential strain and global longitudinal strain were significantly associated with long-term outcome after CRT and had additive prognostic value to routine clinical and electrocardiographic selection criteria for CRT [27]. As it seems from the mentioned studies and from other studies, there is no specific type of strain that is the ultimate one that may evaluate dyssynchrony before CRT implantation and to predict the response to CRT. Furthermore, specific types of strains or combinations of strains but not all types of strains were useful in other conditions. For example, Zhang et al. reported global longitudinal but not circumferential or radial strain predicted prolonged hospitalization and the requirement for inotropic support with epinephrine after aortic valve replacement [23].

In this study, we suggest another model of mechanical dyssynchrony longitudinal rotation that can be easily detected by speckle-tracking echocardiography in addition to the well-known longitudinal, circumferential, and radial strains measured by the same technique. In longitudinal rotation, the SAX-MV (short axis—mitral valve level) algorithm instead of apical views algorithms was selected for analysis. The "posterior" segment (representing the mitral valve) had to be excluded before finalizing the analysis. This unique rotation was not found to be associated with low ejection fraction or the presence of regional wall abnormality or the echocardiography machine used. It may be used alone or in combination with other well-known types of strains to better understand the mechanism of dyssynchrony pre- and post-CRT implantation. Our study is in agreement with the study of Popovic' et al. [11] that showed clockwise longitudinal rotation appeared in the setting of non-ischemic dilated cardiomyopathy with the additional impact of QRS duration. In addition, Popovic' et al. concluded longitudinal rotation was a moderately strong predictor of end systolic volume decrease during CRT in dilated cardiomyopathy. However, the strain-imaging methodology is still undergoing development, and further clinical trials are needed to determine if clinical decisions based on strain imaging result in better outcome [28–30].

4.3. Clinical Outlook

The clinical implication of the longitudinal rotation is not known. However, based on our study and the study of Popovic' et al., this unique and novel method may serve as a simple and reproducible method using speckle-tracking echocardiography with simple modification for finding out optimal candidates for CRT (those who have significant clockwise rotation) and to optimize CRT after implantation by searching for the optimal V-V interval and the optimal left ventricular lead configuration.

4.4. Limitations

This is a small study dealing with the longitudinal rotation of left ventricle. The small number of patients limited the statistical power of ROC analysis and regression analysis. The three groups of patients are not homogeneous. Ejection fraction was lower among the CLBBB group compared to the normal QRS group and the CRBBB group. In addition, left ventricular end diastolic diameter and left ventricular end systolic diameter were larger among the CLBBB patients compared to the normal QRS and CRBBB patients. These differences can be partially explained by the fact that CLBBB (compared to normal QRS and CRBBB) can cause inter- and intra-ventricular dyssynchrony that may result in systolic and diastolic dysfunction and increases in cardiac dimensions. In addition, regional wall motion abnormalities were more common among CLBBB patients compared to normal QRS patients and tended to be more common among CRBBB patients compared to normal QRS patients. However, we found the angle of rotation was not associated with low ejection fraction or the presence of regional wall abnormality.

The clinical significance of this method is not addressed in this study. Thus, clinical inferences cannot be derived from this study. Larger studies are needed to validate this method and to investigate if it would help in predicting responses to CRT or help in optimizing CRT post-implantation beyond the well-known methods.

5. Conclusions

Significant clockwise longitudinal rotation was found in CLBBB patients compared to normal QRS or CRBBB patients using speckle-tracking echocardiography. The angle of this clockwise longitudinal rotation correlated with QRS duration but was not associated with low ejection fraction or the presence of regional wall abnormality or the echocardiography machine used.

Author Contributions: Conceptualization, I.M., R.H., N.A. and S.C.; Methodology, I.M., N.A., S.C., R.H. and Y.H.; Software, I.M., S.C., Y.H. and W.K.; Validation, I.M., W.K., E.B. and S.C.; Formal analysis, I.M., R.H., S.C. and N.A.; Investigation, I.M., R.H., S.C. and Y.H.; Resources, I.M., E.B., S.C. and W.K.; Data curation, R.H., I.M., S.C. and N.A.; Writing—original draft, I.M., R.H., E.B. and S.C.; Writing—review & editing, I.M., E.B., B.M.K. and S.C.; Visualization, I.M., E.B. and S.C.; Supervision, I.M., W.K., E.B. and S.C; Project administration, I.M., R.H., S.C. and Y.H.; Funding acquisition. All authors have read and agreed to the published version of the manuscript.

Funding: This research received no external funding.

Institutional Review Board Statement: The study was conducted in accordance with the Declaration of Helsinki, and approved by the Institutional Ethics Committee of Poriya Medical Center, ethic code: 0099-14-POR.

Informed Consent Statement: Patient consent was waived due to the retrospective design of the study.

Data Availability Statement: Data is unavailable due to privacy or ethical restrictions.

Conflicts of Interest: The authors declare no conflict of interest.

References

1. Kashani, A.; Barold, S.S. Significance of QRS Complex Duration in Patients with Heart Failure. *J. Am. Coll. Cardiol.* **2005**, *46*, 2183–2192. [CrossRef]
2. Bax, J.J.; Ansalone, G.; Breithardt, O.A.; Derumeaux, G.; Leclercq, C.; Schalij, M.J.; Sogaard, P.; John Sutton, M.S.; Petros Nihoyannopoulos MD, FRCP, FACC. Echocardiographic evaluation of cardiac resynchronization therapy: Ready for routine clinical use? A critical appraisal. *J. Am. Coll. Cardiol.* **2004**, *44*, 1–9. [CrossRef]

3. Pitzalis, M.V.; Iacoviello, M.; Romito, R.; Massari, F.; Rizzon, B.; Luzzi, G.; Guida, P.; Andriani, A.; Mastropasqua, F.; Rizzon, P. Cardiac resynchronization therapy tailored by echocardiographic evaluation of ventricular asynchrony. *J. Am. Coll. Cardiol.* **2002**, *40*, 1615–1622. [CrossRef]
4. Yu, C.-M.; Fung, J.W.-H.; Zhang, Q.; Chan, C.-K.; Chan, Y.-S.; Lin, H.; Kum, L.C.; Kong, S.-L.; Zhang, Y.; Sanderson, J.E.; et al. Tissue Doppler Imaging Is Superior to Strain Rate Imaging and Postsystolic Shortening on the Prediction of Reverse Remodeling in Both Ischemic and Nonischemic Heart Failure After Cardiac Resynchronization Therapy. *Circulation* **2004**, *110*, 66–73. [CrossRef]
5. Yu, C.-M.; Chau, E.; Sanderson, J.E.; Fan, K.; Tang, M.-O.; Fung, W.-H.; Lin, H.; Kong, S.-L.; Lam, Y.-M.; Hill, M.R.; et al. Tissue Doppler Echocardiographic Evidence of Reverse Remodeling and Improved Synchronicity by Simultaneously Delaying Regional Contraction After Biventricular Pacing Therapy in Heart Failure. *Circulation* **2002**, *105*, 438–445. [CrossRef]
6. Søgaard, P.; Egeblad, H.; Kim, W.Y.; Jensen, H.K.; Pedersen, A.K.; Kristensen, B.Ø.; Mortensen, P.T. Tissue Doppler imaging predicts improved systolic performance and reversed left ventricular remodeling during long-term cardiac resynchronization therapy. *J. Am. Coll. Cardiol.* **2002**, *40*, 723–730. [CrossRef]
7. Van Bommel, R.J.; Ypenburg, C.; Borleffs, C.J.; Delgado, V.; Marsan, N.A.; Bertini, M.; Holman, E.R.; Schalij, M.J.; Bax, J.J. Value of tissue Doppler echocardiography in predicting response to cardiac resynchronization therapy in patients with heart failure. *Am. J. Cardiol.* **2010**, *105*, 1153–1158. [CrossRef]
8. Gorcsan, J., III; Tanabe, M.; Bleeker, G.B.; Suffoletto, M.S.; Thomas, N.C.; Saba, S.; Tops, L.F.; Schalij, M.J.; Bax, J.J. Combined longitudinal and radial dyssynchrony predicts ventricular response after resynchronization therapy. *J. Am. Coll. Cardiol.* **2007**, *50*, 1476–1483. [CrossRef]
9. Yu, C.M.; Gorcsan, J., III; Bleeker, G.B.; Zhang, Q.; Schalij, M.J.; Suffoletto, M.S.; Fung, J.W.; Schwartzman, D.; Chan, Y.S.; Tanabe, M.; et al. Usefulness of tissue Doppler velocity and strain dyssynchrony for predicting left ventricular reverse remodeling response after cardiac resynchronization therapy. *Am. J. Cardiol.* **2007**, *100*, 1263–1270. [CrossRef]
10. Carasso, S.; Rakowski, H.; Witte, K.K.; Smith, P.; Carasso, D.; Garceau, P.; Sasson, Z.; Parker, J.D. Left ventricular strain patterns in dilated cardiomyopathy predict response to cardiac resynchronization therapy: Timing is not everything. *J. Am. Soc. Echocardiogr.* **2009**, *22*, 242–250. [CrossRef]
11. Popovic, Z.; A Grimm, R.; Ahmad, A.; Agler, D.; Favia, M.; Dan, G.; Lim, P.; Casas, F.; Greenberg, N.L.; Thomas, J.D. Longitudinal rotation: An unrecognised motion pattern in patients with dilated cardiomyopathy. *Heart* **2008**, *94*, e11. [CrossRef]
12. Lang, R.M.; Badano, L.P.; Mor-Avi, V.; Afilalo, J.; Armstrong, A.; Ernande, L.; Flachskampf, F.A.; Foster, E.; Goldstein, S.A.; Kuznetsova, T.; et al. Recommendations for Cardiac Chamber Quantification by Echocardiography in Adults: An Update from the American Society of Echocardiography and the European Association of Cardiovascular Imaging. *J. Am. Soc. Echocardiogr.* **2015**, *28*, 1–39.e14. [CrossRef]
13. Cameli, M.; Mandoli, G.E.; Sciaccaluga, C.; Mondillo, S. More than 10 years of speckle tracking echocardiography: Still a novel technique or a definite tool for clinical practice? *Echocardiography* **2019**, *36*, 958–970. [CrossRef]
14. Rao, H.B.; Krishnaswami, R.; Kalavakolanu, S.; Calambur, N. Ventricular dyssynchrony patterns in left bundle branch block, with and without heart failure. *Indian Pacing Electrophysiol. J.* **2010**, *10*, 115–121.
15. Risum, N.; Jons, C.; Olsen, N.T.; Fritz-Hansen, T.; Bruun, N.E.; Hojgaard, M.V.; Valeur, N.; Kronborg, M.B.; Kisslo, J.; Sogaard, P. Simple regional strain pattern analysis to predict response to cardiac resynchronization therapy: Rationale, initial results, and advantages. *Am. Heart J.* **2012**, *163*, 697–704. [CrossRef]
16. Risum, N.; Tayal, B.; Hansen, T.F.; Bruun, N.E.; Jensen, M.T.; Lauridsen, T.K.; Saba, S.; Kisslo, J.; Gorcsan, J.; Sogaard, P. Identification of Typical Left Bundle Branch Block Contraction by Strain Echocardiography Is Additive to Electrocardiography in Prediction of Long-Term Outcome After Cardiac Resynchronization Therapy. *J. Am. Coll. Cardiol.* **2015**, *66*, 631–641. [CrossRef]
17. Emerek, K.; Friedman, D.J.; Sørensen, P.L.; Hansen, S.M.; Larsen, J.M.; Risum, N.; Thøgersen, A.M.; Graff, C.; Atwater, B.D.; Kisslo, J.; et al. The Association of a classical left bundle Branch Block Contraction Pattern by vendor-independent strain echocardiography and outcome after cardiac resynchronization therapy. *Cardiovasc. Ultrasound* **2019**, *17*, 10. [CrossRef]
18. Calle, S.; Kamoen, V.; De Buyzere, M.; De Pooter, J.; Timmermans, F. A Strain-Based Staging Classification of Left Bundle Branch Block-Induced Cardiac Remodeling. *JACC Cardiovasc. Imaging* **2021**, *14*, 1691–1702. [CrossRef]
19. Eriksson, J.; Zajac, J.; Alehagen, U.; Bolger, A.F.; Ebbers, T.; Carlhäll, C.-J. Left ventricular hemodynamic forces as a marker of mechanical dyssynchrony in heart failure patients with left bundle branch block. *Sci. Rep.* **2017**, *7*, 2971. [CrossRef]
20. Khan, F.Z.; Virdee, M.S.; Palmer, C.R.; Pugh, P.J.; O'Halloran, D.; Elsik, M.; Read, P.A.; Begley, D.; Fynn, S.P.; Dutka, D.P. Targeted Left Ventricular Lead Placement to Guide Cardiac Resynchronization Therapy: The TARGET Study: A Randomized, Controlled Trial. *J. Am. Coll. Cardiol.* **2012**, *59*, 1509–1518. [CrossRef]
21. Sommer, A.; Kronborg, M.B.; Nørgaard, B.L.; Poulsen, S.H.; Bouchelouche, K.; Böttcher, M.; Jensen, H.K.; Jensen, J.M.; Kristensen, J.; Gerdes, C.; et al. Multimodality imaging-guided left ventricular lead placement in cardiac resynchronization therapy: A randomized controlled trial. *Eur. J. Heart Fail.* **2016**, *18*, 1365–1374. [CrossRef]
22. Lunati, M.; Magenta, G.; Cattafi, G.; Moreo, A.; Falaschi, G.; Contardi, D.; Locati, E. Clinical Relevance of Systematic CRT Device Optimization. *J. Atr. Fibrillation* **2014**, *7*, 1077.
23. Zhang, K.; Sheu, R.; Zimmerman, N.M.; Alfirevic, A.; Sale, S.; Gillinov, A.M.; Duncan, A.E. A Comparison of Global Longitudinal, Circumferential, and Radial Strain to Predict Outcomes After Cardiac Surgery. *J. Cardiothorac. Vasc. Anesthesia* **2019**, *33*, 1315–1322. [CrossRef]

24. Delgado, V.; Ypenburg, C.; van Bommel, R.J.; Tops, L.F.; Mollema, S.A.; Marsan, N.A.; Bleeker, G.B.; Schalij, M.J.; Bax, J.J. Assessment of Left Ventricular Dyssynchrony by Speckle Tracking Strain Imaging: Comparison Between Longitudinal, Circumferential, and Radial Strain in Cardiac Resynchronization Therapy. *J. Am. Coll. Cardiol.* **2008**, *51*, 1944–1952. [CrossRef]
25. Helm, R.H.; Leclercq, C.; Faris, O.P.; Ozturk, C.; McVeigh, E.; Lardo, A.; Kass, D.A. Cardiac dyssynchrony analysis using circumferential versus longitudinal strain: Implications for assessing cardiac resynchronization. *Circulation* **2005**, *111*, 2760–2767. [CrossRef]
26. Wang, C.-L.; Wu, C.-T.; Yeh, Y.-H.; Wu, L.-S.; Chan, Y.-H.; Kuo, C.-T.; Chu, P.-H.; Hsu, L.-A.; Ho, W.-J. Left bundle-branch block contraction patterns identified from radial-strain analysis predicts outcomes following cardiac resynchronization therapy. *Int. J. Cardiovasc. Imaging* **2017**, *33*, 869–877. [CrossRef]
27. Delgado-Montero, A.; Tayal, B.; Goda, A.; Ryo, K.; Marek, J.J.; Sugahara, M.; Qi, Z.; Althouse, A.D.; Saba, S.; Schwartzman, D.; et al. Additive Prognostic Value of Echocardiographic Global Longitudinal and Global Circumferential Strain to Electrocardiographic Criteria in Patients with Heart Failure Undergoing Cardiac Resynchronization Therapy. *Circ. Cardiovasc. Imaging* **2016**, *9*, e004241. [CrossRef]
28. Smiseth, O.A.; Torp, H.; Opdahl, A.; Haugaa, K.H.; Urheim, S. Myocardial strain imaging: How useful is it in clinical decision making? *Eur. Heart J.* **2016**, *37*, 1196–1207. [CrossRef]
29. Olsen, F.J.; Biering-Sørensen, T. Myocardial Strain and Dyssynchrony: Incremental Value? *Heart Fail. Clin.* **2019**, *15*, 167–178. [CrossRef]
30. Sareen, N.; Ananthasubramaniam, K. Strain Imaging: From Physiology to Practical Applications in Daily Practice. *Cardiol. Rev.* **2016**, *24*, 56–69. [CrossRef]

Disclaimer/Publisher's Note: The statements, opinions and data contained in all publications are solely those of the individual author(s) and contributor(s) and not of MDPI and/or the editor(s). MDPI and/or the editor(s) disclaim responsibility for any injury to people or property resulting from any ideas, methods, instructions or products referred to in the content.

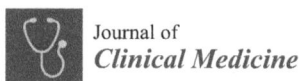
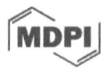

Article

Long-Term Outcomes of Tachycardia-Induced Cardiomyopathy Compared with Idiopathic Dilated Cardiomyopathy

Moshe Katz [1,2,3,*], Amit Meitus [2], Michael Arad [1,2], Anthony Aizer [3], Eyal Nof [1,2] and Roy Beinart [1,2]

[1] Sheba Medical Center, Ramat Gan 5266202, Israel
[2] Sackler School of Medicine, Tel-Aviv University, Tel Aviv 6997801, Israel
[3] NYU Grossman School of Medicine, New York, NY 10016, USA
* Correspondence: moshe.katz@nyulangone.org; Tel.: +1-914-893-7914

Abstract: Background: data on the natural course and prognosis of tachycardia-induced cardiomyopathy (TICMP) and comparison with idiopathic dilated cardiomyopathies (IDCM) are scarce. Objective: To compare the clinical presentation, comorbidities, and long-term outcomes of TICMP patients with IDCM patients. Methods: a retrospective cohort study of patients hospitalized with new-onset TICMP or IDCM. The primary endpoint was a composite of death, myocardial infarction, thromboembolic events, assist device, heart transplantation, and ventricular tachycardia or fibrillation (VT/VF). The secondary endpoint was recurrent hospitalization due to heart failure (HF) exacerbation. Results: the cohort was comprised of 64 TICMP and 66 IDCM patients. The primary composite endpoint and all-cause mortality were similar between the groups during a median follow-up of ~6 years (36% versus 29%, $p = 0.33$ and 22% versus 15%, $p = 0.15$, respectively). Survival analysis showed no significant difference between TICMP and IDCM groups for the composite endpoint ($p = 0.75$), all-cause mortality ($p = 0.65$), and hospitalizations due to heart failure exacerbation. Nonetheless, the incidence of recurrent hospitalization was significantly higher in TICMP patients (incidence rate ratio 1.59; $p = 0.009$). Conclusions: patients with TICMP have similar long-term outcomes as those with IDCM. However, it portends a higher rate of HF readmissions, mostly due to arrhythmia recurrences.

Keywords: arrhythmia; cardiomyopathy; atrial fibrillation; heart failure; premature ventricular beats

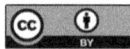

1. Introduction

Tachycardia-induced cardiomyopathy (TICMP), also known as arrhythmia-induced cardiomyopathy (AIC), is a subtype of acquired dilated cardiomyopathy [1]. TICMP has been documented in different forms of arrhythmia, including supraventricular tachycardia (SVT), atrial tachycardia (AT), ventricular tachycardia (VT), and frequent premature ventricular beats (PVBs), but most frequently it has been recognized in patients with atrial fibrillation (AF) and atrial flutter (AFL) [2].

TICMP is often considered a relatively benign cause of heart failure, and reversible when appropriate treatments are given in a timely fashion [3,4]. Treatment strategies mainly focus on rhythm control, following cardioversion and medication or ablation procedure, though rate control may also be implemented [5,6].

Short-term outcomes post-treatment usually demonstrate improvement in the left ventricular ejection fraction (LVEF) and left ventricular dimensions [7]. Notably, several studies reported an increased risk of sudden cardiac death, even following improvement in LV function [8,9]. However, data on the long-term outcomes of TICMP patients are lacking [9,10]. Both TICMP and IDCM are characterized by ventricular dilatation and depressed LV function and should be considered after ruling out hypertension, valvular, congenital, or ischemic heart disease [11]. They differ in etiology, baseline echocardiographic parameters, and reversibility of left ventricular systolic function with treatment. Yet, the prognosis and outcomes of these entities are unclear.

Objective: to compare the clinical presentation, comorbidities, and long-term outcomes of TICMP patients with IDCM patients.

2. Methods

2.1. Study Population

The study is a retrospective cohort analysis, aimed at comparing the prognosis of TICMP (n = 64) with IDCM (n = 66) patients. All electronic medical records of patients admitted to the Sheba Medical Center for heart failure and cardiomyopathy between March 2007 and June 2017 were enrolled. The etiologies causing heart failure or cardiomyopathy were defined. This initial database included subjects with new-onset cardiomyopathy. All patients were ≥18 years old and with LVEF ≤ 50% at presentation. Patients were defined as IDCM in the absence of any of the following conditions: ischemia, uncontrolled hypertension (>160/100), severe valvular disease, congenital heart disease, toxic exposure (chemotherapy/alcohol consumption, etc.), metabolic etiologies (nutritional deficiencies, endocrinopathy, etc.), or tachyarrhythmia. Patients were defined as TICMP if presented with heart failure secondary to arrhythmia without any other apparent causes for cardiomyopathy, and also showed an improvement of at least 15% in LVEF after rhythm control or rate control [12] within 6 months.

Once the cohort was established, a thorough investigation of each patient record was performed using the Sheba Medical Center computerized medical records. Demographic and clinical data and diagnostic imaging studies were collected and analyzed. In addition, the death date was retrieved from governmental mortality records.

During the index hospitalization, patients received guidelines-based therapy for heart failure, including angiotensin-converting enzyme inhibitors or angiotensin receptor blockers, beta-blockers, aldosterone receptor antagonists, digitalis, and diuretics if needed. In addition, patients with TICMP were treated with rhythm control or rate control strategies according to physicians' discretion.

2.2. Study End Points

The primary endpoint was a composite of death, myocardial infarction, thromboembolic events, assist device, heart transplantation, and symptomatic VT/VF. The secondary endpoint was recurrent hospitalization due to heart failure exacerbation.

Study endpoints were evaluated at 5 years and for the whole length follow-up.

The Institutional Review Board of Sheba Medical Center approved this study.

2.3. Statistical Analysis

Comparisons between groups were analyzed by Chi-square or Fisher's exact tests for categorical parameters, and Mann–Whitney test for continuous parameters. The non-normally distributed continuous variables were reported as a median and interquartile range [Q1–Q3]. Categorical variables were reported as numbers and percentages. The length of follow-up was described using the reverse censoring method. Kaplan–Meier curves were used to describe time to the primary endpoint, as well as recurrent hospitalization due to heart failure exacerbation. A log-rank test was used to compare survival between groups. Cox regression was done to estimate the crude hazard ratio for the primary and secondary endpoints. A propensity score was used to reduce the effects of confounding in the baseline characteristic between study groups. The propensity score for an individual is defined as the probability of being assigned to TICMP given all relevant covariates. The propensity score was calculated using logistic regression and then stratified into quintiles. The following variables were used to calculate the propensity score: age, sex, hypertension, smoking, cerebrovascular disease, diabetes mellitus, diabetes mellitus treated with insulin, peripheral vascular disease, valvular heart disease, ischemic heart disease, and LVEF.

To reduce the effect of confounders, stratified cox regression by the propensity score quintiles was performed for the primary and secondary endpoint. To compare the incidence of recurrent hospitalization during the follow-up period, Poisson regression was applied to estimate the incidence rate ratio. The natural logarithm of the length of follow-up was used as an offset variable in the Poisson model.

All statistical tests were two-tailed. $p < 0.05$ was considered statistically significant.

SPSS software was used for statistical analysis (IBM SPSS Statistics, Version 25, IBM Corp, Armonk, NY, USA, 2017).

3. Results

Sixty-four TICMP and 66 IDCM patients were hospitalized at the Sheba Medical Center with new onset heart failure between March 2007 and June 2017 (Figure 1). Baseline demographic characteristics and co-morbidities of the study population are shown in Table 1. In both groups, patients were predominantly males, overweight, and with a significant proportion of pre-existing hypertension. Patients in the TICMP group had a higher proportion of preexisting non-significant valvular heart disease (11% versus 2%, $p = 0.03$). There were no other significant differences in demographics and medical history. The most common etiology for TICMP was atrial fibrillation (76%), of whom 17 (27%) had a history of atrial fibrillation prior to admission (Table S1).

Clinical characteristics: vital signs, NYHA function class, and echocardiographic and electrocardiographic findings, performed upon presentation, are shown in Table 2. Overall, patients in both groups presented with similar severity of symptoms, as evidenced by the NYHA function class. As expected, heart rates were much faster in TICMP patients, with a median heart rate of 120 bpm [IQR 90–132] versus 82 bpm [IQR 73–103] in idiopathic DCM patients ($p < 0.001$). There were no significant differences in laboratory study results. Prescription drug data showed higher use of beta-blockers prior to admission in the TICMP group compared with that of IDCM (55% versus 17%, $p < 0.001$). Anti-arrhythmic drug use was also higher in TICMP patients (20% versus 3%, $p = 0.002$), as well as statin use (41% versus 21%, $p = 0.02$).

Table 1. Baseline demographic characteristics and co-morbidities.

	IDCM N = 66	TICMP N = 64	p-Value
Sex, male; n (%)	51 (77)	41 (64)	0.1
Age, years; median [IQR]	60 [47–69]	65 [57–69]	0.09
BMI, kg/m^2; median [IQR]	29 [24–33]	29 [26–33]	0.36
Hypertension, mmHg; n (%)	33 (50)	32 (50)	1
Current smoker; n (%)	15 (23)	7 (11)	0.08
CVD; n (%)	6 (9)	9 (14)	0.38
DM; n (%)	13 (20)	12 (19)	0.89
DM insulin Tx; n (%)	3 (5)	2 (3)	0.67
PVD; n (%)	6 (9)	3 (5)	0.49
VHD; n (%)	1 (2)	7 (11)	0.03 *
IHD; n (%)	6 (9)	5 (8)	0.79

BMI—body mass index; CVD—cerebrovascular disease; DM—diabetes mellitus; IDCM—idiopathic dilated cardiomyopathy; IHD—ischemic heart disease; IQR—interquartile range; PVD—peripheral vascular disease; TICMP—tachycardia-induced cardiomyopathy Tx-therapy; VHD—valvular heart disease. Chi-square or Fisher's exact tests were performed for categorical parameters. Mann–Whitney test was performed for continuous parameters. Significant p-value was marked by *.

Table 2. Clinical characteristics at presentation.

	IDCM N = 66	TICMP N = 64	p-Value
Heart rate, BPM; median [IQR]	82 [73–103]	120 [90–132]	<0.001 *
SBP, mmHg; median [IQR]	132 [120–144]	127 [117–139]	0.16
DBP, mmHg; median [IQR]	75 [67–93]	83 [70–92]	0.44
NYHA FC; n (%)			
I	2 (3)	2 (3)	
II	25 (39)	30 (47)	0.34
III	26 (40)	27 (42)	
IV	12 (18)	5 (8)	
Laboratory results			
LDL, mg/dL; median [IQR]	105 [87–133]	105 [86–127]	0.7
HDL, mg/dL; median [IQR]	38 [32–46]	40 [32–47]	0.86
Triglycerides, mg/dL; median [IQR]	109 [77–150]	104 [74–147]	0.54
HGB, g/dL; median [IQR]	13.7 [12.5–14.8]	13.6 [12.5–14.6]	0.68
TSH, mIU/L; median [IQR]	1.8 [1.26–2.6]	1.95 [1.37–3.18]	0.47
Creatinine, mg/dL; median [IQR]	1.04 [0.88–1.25]	1.05 [0.89–1.26]	0.62
Albumin, g/dL; median [IQR]	3.9 [3.7–4.2]	3.8 [3.6–4]	0.06
Medical treatment			
Beta-blockers; n (%)	11 (17)	35 (55)	<0.001 *
CCBs; n (%)	5 (8)	5 (8)	0.96
Statins; n (%)	14 (21)	26 (41)	0.02 *
ACE inhibitors; n (%)	12 (18)	16 (25)	0.34
ARBs; n (%)	6 (9)	11 (17)	0.17
Digitalis; n (%)	0	1 (3)	0.24
AADs; n (%)	2 (3)	13 (20)	0.002 *
Echocardiography			
LVEF, %; median [IQR]	25 [15–35]	30 [20–32]	0.11
LVEDD, cm; median [IQR]	5.8 [5.5–6.4]	5.1 [4.6–5.6]	<0.001 *
LVESD, cm; median [IQR]	5 [4.5–6.2]	3.8 [3.5–4.9]	<0.001 *
LA diameter, cm; median [IQR]	4.6 [4.1–4.8]	4.5 [4.2–4.8]	0.98
LV mass, g; median [IQR]	231 [206–268]	195 [158–242]	<0.001 *
SPAP, mmHg; median [IQR]	42 [32–50]	40 [35–46]	0.8
Electrocardiography			
QRS duration, ms; median [IQR]	106 [96–148]	98 [86–111]	0.002 *
LBBB; n (%)	21 (32)	7 (11)	0.003 *
RBBB; n (%)	2 (3)	6 (10)	0.13
PR interval, ms; median [IQR]	158 [138–174]	174 [150–192]	0.003 *
QTc, ms; median [IQR]	475 [452–501]	467 [436–491]	0.17

AADs—antiarrhythmic drugs; ACE—angiotensin-converting enzyme; ARBs—angiotensin II receptor blockers; BPM—beats per minute; CCBs—calcium channel blockers; DBP—diastolic blood pressure; HDL—high-density lipoprotein; HGB—hemoglobin; IDCM—idiopathic dilated cardiomyopathy; LA—left atrium; LDL—low-density lipoprotein; LVEDD—left ventricular end-diastolic diameter; LVEF—left ventricular ejection fraction; LVESD—left ventricular end-systolic diameter; NYHA FC—New York Heart Association Functional Classification; IQR—interquartile range; SBP—systolic blood pressure; SPAP—systolic pulmonary artery pressure TICMP—tachycardia-induced cardiomyopathy; TSH—thyroid-stimulating hormone. Chi-square or Fisher's exact tests were performed for categorical parameters. Mann–Whitney test was performed for continuous parameters. Significant p-value was marked by *.

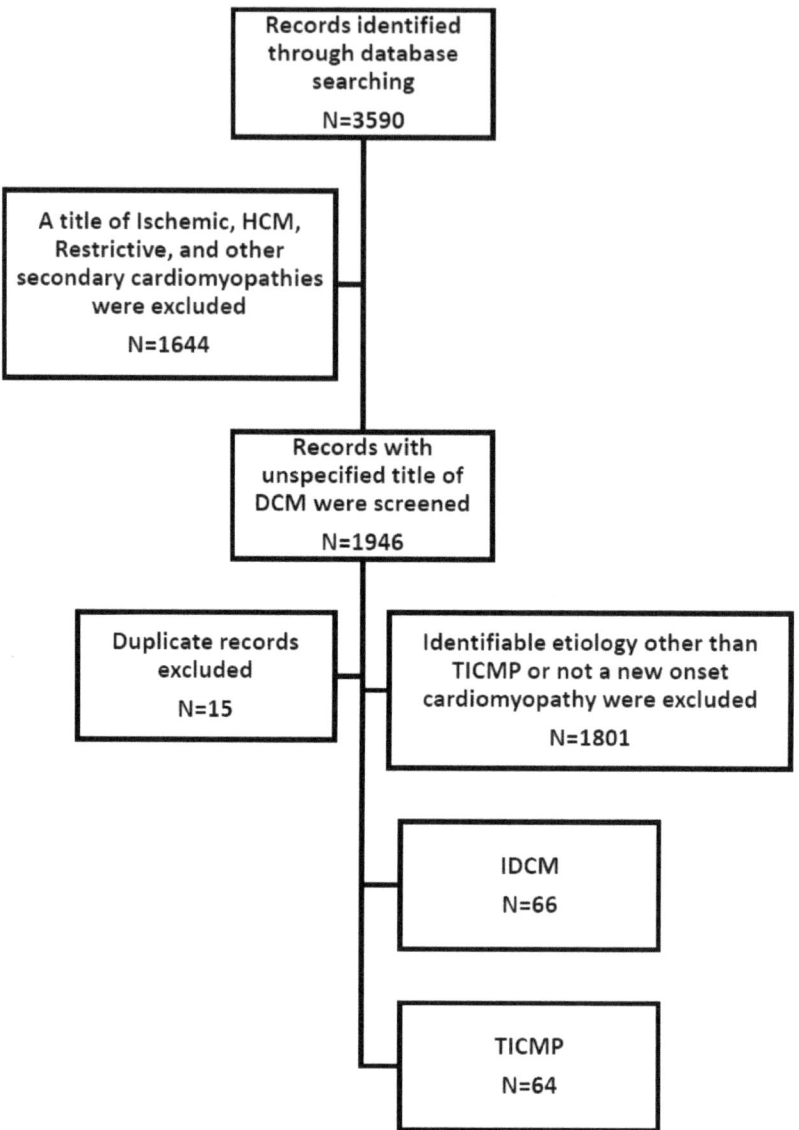

Figure 1. Flow chart of study population. DCM—dilated cardiomyopathy; HCM—hypertrophic cardiomyopathy; IDCM—idiopathic dilated cardiomyopathy; TICMP—tachycardia-induced cardiomyopathy.

Echocardiographic findings demonstrated, as expected, significant differences in left ventricle dimensions, with IDCM patients having larger dimensions. The left ventricular end-diastolic diameter in IDCM was 5.8 cm [5.5–6.4] versus 5.1 cm [4.6–5.6] in TICMP, $p < 0.001$, and left ventricular end-systolic diameter in IDCM was 5 cm [4.5–6.2] versus 3.8 cm [3.5–4.9] in TICMP, $p < 0.001$. Similarly, left ventricle mass was significantly higher in IDCM patients (231 g [206–268] versus 195 g [158–242], $p < 0.001$).

As for electrocardiographic findings, IDCM patients had a more frequent left bundle branch block pattern (32% versus 11%, $p = 0.003$). The QRS duration was also significantly longer compared with those of TICMP patients (106 ms [96–148] versus 98 ms [86–111],

p = 0.002). Prolonged QRS duration (QRS duration equal to or greater than 110 milliseconds) was found in 26 IDCM patients versus 18 TICMP patients. However, the difference was not statistically significant. Interestingly, the PR interval was longer in TICMP patients, albeit within the normal range (174 ms [150–192] versus 158 ms [138–174], p = 0.003).

Overall coronary artery disease assessment, including invasive coronary angiography, coronary computed tomography angiography (CCTA), ergometry, and/or single photon emission computed tomography (SPECT) was performed in 64 (97%) IDCM patients and 53 (83%) TICMP patients, p = 0.007. Two patients (3%) in IDCM did not have an ischemic workup in our institution. One had an ischemic evaluation in a different institution and was lost to follow-up. His parameters were mainly used for baseline characteristics. The second had severe chronic kidney disease and refused ischemic evaluation.

During the index hospitalization, only 5 (8%) patients with IDCM presented with arrhythmia as a secondary finding rather than the cause for cardiomyopathy. For TICMP patients, a rhythm control strategy was chosen in 51 (80%) patients. The remaining were treated with rate control. Four of these were treated with pacemaker (PM) implantation as part of the pace and ablate strategy, two single-chamber PMs, and two cardiac resynchronization therapy pacemakers (CRTP).

Follow-up: data were typically obtained for all patients 3 to 6 months following discharge. The median LVEF during follow-up was much lower in IDCM compared with TICMP patients (35% [IQR 20–45%], 55% [IQR 47–60%], respectively, p < 0.001). LVEF improved during follow-up in both groups (Table S2), however, TICMP patients had greater improvement with a median improvement of 25% [IQR 18–30%] compared with only 9% [IQR 5–15%] in IDCM (p < 0.001). During follow-up, more TICMP patients underwent pacemaker implantation (12 versus 1, p = 0.001): 10 out of 12 (83%) pacemakers were implanted as part of pace and ablate strategy (three CRTP, three dual-chamber PMs, and four single chamber PMs), and two dual chamber pacemakers for advanced atrioventricular block (AVB) and sick sinus syndrome. As expected, fewer TICMP patients were implanted with intracardiac defibrillators (5% versus 35%, p < 0.001) because the left ventricular ejection fraction recovered over time. Three TICMP patients underwent implantable cardioverter defibrillator (ICD) implantation during follow-up. One patient had very long QT with uncontrolled frequent premature ventricular beats and underwent dual chamber ICD implantation due to a high risk of Torsades de Pointes (TdP). The second patient underwent cardiac resynchronization therapy defibrillator (CRTD) implantation due to episodes of long short sequences leading to non-sustained TdP. The third patient underwent dual chamber ICD for secondary prevention after experiencing myocardial infarction and sustained ventricular tachycardia. Fourteen IDCM patients underwent CRTD implantation. Ten out of the fourteen patients who were implanted with CRTD had left bundle branch block (LBBB) at presentation.

Study Endpoints

The primary composite endpoint and all-cause mortality were similar between TICMP and IDCM groups during a median follow-up time of 6.43 years [IQR 5.2–8.2]. During the follow-up, 24 of 130 (18%) patients died, 10 (15%) in the IDCM group and 14 (22%) in the TICMP group (Table 3). A Kaplan–Meier survival analysis showed no significant difference between TICMP and IDCM groups for event-free survival of the composite endpoint (log rank, p = 0.328) and all-cause mortality (Log Rank, p = 0.139) (Figures 2 and 3). In univariate analysis, the mean time to readmission for heart failure exacerbation was shorter in the TICMP patients 5.2 years (95% CI 4–6.4) versus 6.9 years (95% CI 5.9–8) (log rank, p = 0.035) (Figure 4). However, this difference became statistically insignificant in multivariate analysis following propensity score adjustment (HR: 1.55; 95% CI 0.85–2.8; p = 0.15) (Table 4). Interestingly, Poisson regression analysis showed that the incidence of recurrent hospitalizations during the follow-up period was much higher in TICMP patients (incidence rate ratio 1.59, 95% CI 1.12–2.24; p = 0.009). The main trigger for heart failure exacerbation in TICMP patients was arrhythmia recurrence, while exacerbations in IDCM were mainly due to nonadherence to medical advice (Table 5). Nonadherence was defined as forgetting to take medications or skipping doses in the 2 weeks before arriving at the emergency department.

Table 3. Composite outcome events.

	IDCM N = 66	TICMP N = 64	p-Value
All-cause mortality; n (%)	10 (15)	14 (22)	0.37
Acute coronary syndrome; n (%)	4 (6)	4 (6)	1
Thromboembolic events; n (%)	7 (11)	4 (7)	0.39
LVAD/heart transplant; n (%)	1 (2)	0	NA
Symptomatic VT/VF; n (%)	2 (3)	4 (6)	0.44

IDCM—idiopathic dilated cardiomyopathy; LVAD—left ventricular assist device; NA—not applicable; TICMP—tachycardia-induced cardiomyopathy; VT/VF—ventricular tachycardia or ventricular fibrillation. Fisher's exact test was performed for categorical parameters.

Table 4. Crude and adjusted hazard ratios of the study endpoints.

Outcome	Crude		Propensity Score	
	HR 95% CI	p-Value	HR 95% CI	p-Value
Whole follow-up				
Composite endpoint	1.35 (0.74–2.4)	0.33	1.11 (0.57–2.18)	0.75
All-cause mortality	1.84 (0.81–4.17)	0.15	1.25 (0.49–3.17)	0.65
HF hospitalization	1.81 (1.03–3.18)	0.04 *	1.55 (0.85–2.8)	0.15
5 years follow-up				
Composite endpoint	0.97 (0.49–1.93)	0.94	0.84 (0.4–1.75)	0.64
All-cause mortality	1.47 (0.51–4.25)	0.47	1.09 (0.35–3.4)	0.88
HF hospitalization	1.6 (0.87–2.94)	0.13	1.43 (0.75–2.71)	0.28

CI—confidence interval; HF—heart failure. Cox regression was done to estimate the crude hazard ratio for the primary and secondary endpoints. Significant p-value was marked by *.

Table 5. Triggers for 1st heart failure recurrence.

	IDCM n = 21 N = 66	TICMP n = 30 N = 64
No trigger identified; n (%)	5 (8)	2 (3)
AF/AFL; n (%)	1 (2)	22 (34)
Bradyarrhythmia; n (%)	1 (2)	1 (2)
SVT; n (%)	0	1 (2)
Infection; n (%)	3 (5)	1 (2)
Concurrent lung disease; n (%)	1 (2)	0
Nonadherence; n (%)	7 (11)	1 (2)
Acute kidney injury; n (%)	1 (2)	0
Post-surgery volume overload; n (%)	1 (2)	1 (2)
Post-myocardial infarction; n (%)	1 (2)	0
Ventricular tachycardia; n (%)	0	1 (2)

AF—atrial fibrillation; AFL—atrial flutter; IDCM—idiopathic dilated cardiomyopathy; SVT—supraventricular tachycardia; TICMP—tachycardia-induced cardiomyopathy. Twenty-one IDCM patients and thirty TICMP patients had heart failure recurrence during follow-up. Percentages represent the absolute number of heart failure recurrences from the total cohort in each group.

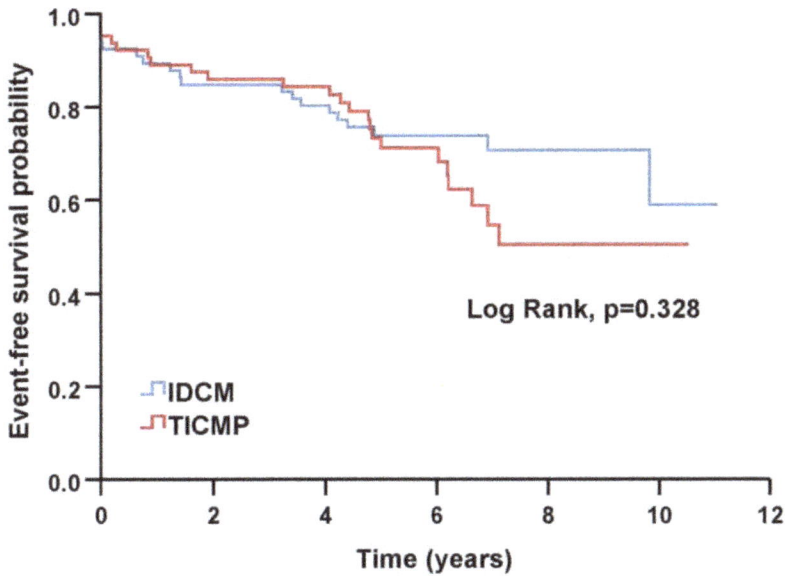

Figure 2. Kaplan–Meier curve of time to primary composite endpoint. IDCM—idiopathic dilated cardiomyopathy; TICMP—tachycardia-induced cardiomyopathy.

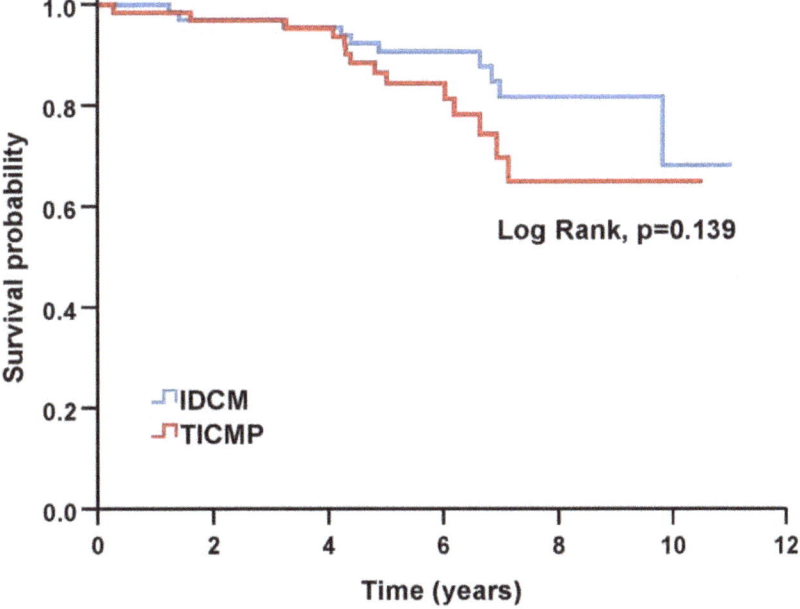

Figure 3. Kaplan–Meier estimates of overall survival based on the type of cardiomyopathy. IDCM—idiopathic dilated cardiomyopathy; TICMP—tachycardia-induced cardiomyopathy.

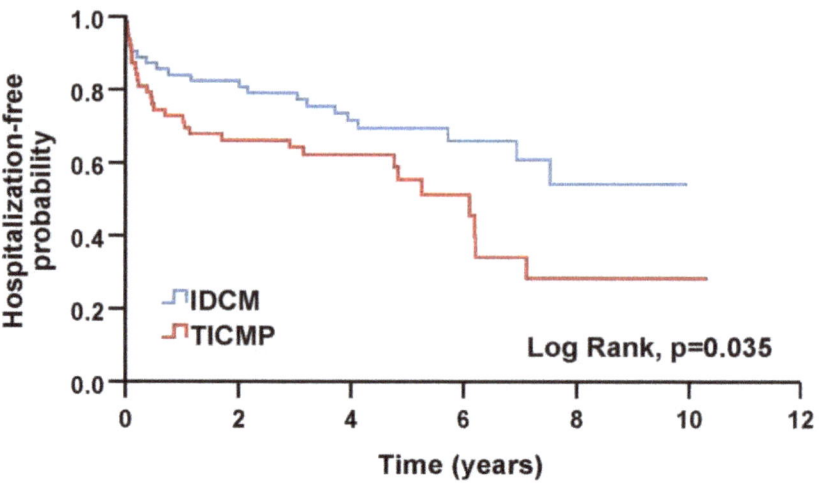

Figure 4. Kaplan–Meier survival probabilities for patients admitted for a first heart failure hospitalization. IDCM—idiopathic dilated cardiomyopathy; TICMP—tachycardia-induced cardiomyopathy.

4. Discussion

In this study, we assessed the clinical presentation and prognosis of TICMP patients and compared them to IDCM patients. The main findings of the present study were: (1) All-cause mortality rates are similar between TICMP and IDCM; (2) The composite endpoint of death, myocardial infarction, thromboembolic events, assist device, heart transplantation, and VT/VF (primary endpoint) are similar between these groups; (3) Similar first readmission due to heart failure exacerbation; (4) Recurrent admission rates are significantly higher in TICMP patients mainly due to arrhythmia recurrences.

Our study represents a relatively large real-world cohort comprised of patients hospitalized with new onset cardiomyopathy (TICMP or IDCM). It adds information to previously published studies on TICMP. These studies, however, included relatively small sample size cohorts, and mainly from patients who underwent catheter ablations, possibly resulting in inherent selection bias [5,10].

Dilated cardiomyopathy belongs to the primary cardiomyopathies, disorders predominantly affecting the heart muscle, and is defined by the presence of left ventricular dilatation and systolic dysfunction in the absence of known abnormal loading conditions or significant coronary artery disease [13,14]. Genetic mutations can be found in up to 35% of dilated cardiomyopathy cases. Non-genetic causes such as drug toxicity, myocarditis, and more may result in similar clinical presentations [15,16]. When an underlying pathology cannot be identified, patients are diagnosed with IDCM [17].

The underlying cause of dilated cardiomyopathy determines the prognosis. Patients with IDCM usually have a better prognosis compared with patients with cardiomyopathy due to infiltrative disease, HIV infection, connective tissue disease, or doxorubicin [18].

TICMP is the result of prolonged and persistent tachycardia, and its prognosis is perceived by clinicians as relatively better. One expects that once the arrhythmia is controlled, recovery of LV function is seen over time. However, prolonged tachycardia results in elevated left ventricular filling pressures, impaired ventricular contractile function, reduced cardiac output, elevated systemic vascular resistance, and increased left ventricular wall stress. These hemodynamic changes lead to upregulation of the neurohormonal axis, which results in cellular and molecular changes. Furthermore, changes may remain even after improvement in the LV function and can serve as an arrhythmogenic substrate for arrhythmia recurrence [19]. In fact, animal models of tachycardia-induced cardiomyopathy demonstrated repolarization abnormalities, QT interval prolongation, polymorphic ventricular tachycardia, and sudden cardiac death. A human study supports these findings and implies a risk of sudden death even after controlling the heart rate and LVEF improvement [8].

In the present study, we found some major differences between IDCM and TICMP patients. These were mainly related to presenting symptoms, electrocardiography, and echocardiography measurements as well as some parameters during follow-up.

We found that the most common arrhythmia resulting in TICMP was atrial fibrillation (76%) (Table S1). In approximately two-thirds of the patients, TICMP was the presenting symptom of atrial fibrillation, while others had a history of this arrhythmia. Not surprisingly, patients with TICMP had faster heart rates at presentation. Indeed, they were treated more with beta-blockers and antiarrhythmic drugs prior to their first admission. This suggests that TICMP can develop over time in patients with a recurrence of atrial fibrillation. Our findings are in keeping with previously published studies [8].

Electrocardiographic parameters were also different between the groups. Patients with IDCM had shorter PR intervals but wider QRS intervals with more frequent left bundle branch block patterns. This may lead by itself to cardiomyopathy or further deteriorate LV dysfunction regardless of the primary cause [20–23]. In this study, approximately 30% of patients with IDCM had LBBB, and half of them were treated with a bi-ventricular defibrillator (10 out of 21 patients). IDCM patients who received a bi-ventricular defibrillator had a small improvement in their ejection fraction after CRTD implantation. This fact strongly supports the diagnosis of IDCM over left bundle branch-mediated cardiomyopathy because in LBBB-mediated cardiomyopathy, the LVEF usually normalizes after CRTD implantation [23]. In addition, our data are in line with previous registry data that found that LBBB is common in patients with heart failure [24]. Vera et al. examined electrocardiogram and cardiac magnetic resonance (CMR) parameters of patients admitted for heart failure with reduced LVEF and concomitant supraventricular tachycardia [25]. Findings were analyzed to predict LVEF recovery. Like our cohort, they found that patients with dilated cardiomyopathy (DCM) had wider QRS than patients with TICMP. On CMR, the TICMP presented with higher LVEF whereas late gadolinium enhancement (LGE) was more frequent in dilated cardiomyopathy. QRS $\geq$ 100 ms, LVEF < 40% on CMR, and the presence of LGE were independent predictors of lack of LVEF recovery. In addition, during follow-up, DCM patients were more frequently admitted for heart failure than TICMP. In contrast to that, the LVEF in our cohort was not statistically different in both groups and we found that patients with TICMP were more frequently admitted for heart failure than DCM. The difference in heart failure re-admissions between studies can be explained by the different definitions of DCM and TICMP in the studies and the differences in presenting LVEF. In our cohort, we included only idiopathic dilated cardiomyopathy and not all patients diagnosed with dilated cardiomyopathy. Patients who have dilated cardiomyopathy secondary to other conditions may have a worse prognosis than patients with idiopathic dilated cardiomyopathy depending on the underlying etiology. Moreover, TICMP was defined as recovery to LVEF above 50% while our definition required an improvement of at least 15% in LVEF after rhythm control or rate control. Consequent to that, our TICMP cohort included patients with LVEF lower than 50% on follow-up (25% of TICMP patients had LVEF less than 47%). Lower LVEF improvement results in more heart failure hospitalizations [26]. The combination of heterogeneity, lower presenting LVEF in the DCM group, and including only TICMP patients with LVEF above 50% on follow-up contributed to the different results in these studies.

Dissimilarities in echocardiography measurements were also noted between the groups. Larger left ventricular dimensions and left ventricular mass were found in patients with IDCM. Jeong et al. reported that the initial echocardiographic parameters, especially the left ventricular end diastolic dimension can help differentiate TICMP from IDCM [12]. Similarly, we found larger left ventricular dimensions; however, there is a substantial overlap between the groups, and distinguishing between them solely based on ECG or echocardiography parameters could be challenging and at times misleading.

Importantly, with appropriate guideline-based medical therapy, including heart failure medications, treatment with antiarrhythmic drugs, or catheter ablation when appropriate, the LVEF increased in both groups. Notably, this improvement was substantially higher in the TICMP group during follow-up.

In terms of prognosis, no differences were found in respect of the primary and secondary endpoints. Hence, both mortality rates and the composite end point of death, myocardial infarction, thromboembolic events, assist device, heart transplantation, and VT/VF were similar between the groups. A possible explanation might be the higher proportion of AF in our cohort, an independent predictor of morbidity and mortality [27]. Hence, the "AF effect" occurring in TICMP patients might counterbalance the improvement in LVEF following appropriate treatment. Surprisingly, despite a high prevalence of AF in the TICMP group, we found similar rates of thromboembolic events in both groups. This could be attributed to both adherence to anticoagulation treatment in patients with AF and high risk for stroke, and a significant improvement in LVEF over time. In contrast, patients with IDCM were not routinely treated with anticoagulation, unless otherwise indicated, and had only slight improvement in LVEF, which can lead to venous stasis and subsequently to the creation of de novo mural thrombi [28]. Interestingly, the risk for first heart failure exacerbation was similar between both groups during the follow-up, although patients with TICMP had higher rates of recurrent HF-related hospitalizations during follow-up. The latter is mainly related to tachyarrhythmia recurrence (Table 5). Ahmad et al. reported a 50% recurrence rate of arrhythmia in patients with TICMP over a median follow-up of 6 months. They found that recurrence of arrhythmia was significantly associated with heart failure hospitalizations with an odds ratio of 6.65. However, after adjusting for other clinical characteristics, this association was not significant [29]. The lack of correlation between arrhythmia recurrence and heart failure hospitalizations in the multivariate analysis may stem from the way they defined arrhythmia recurrence and the clinical setting that it occurred in. Arrhythmia recurrence was based on a premature ventricular burden exceeding 10% or a 30-s episode of atrial fibrillation or atrial flutter during ambulatory monitoring. Therefore, they could have included patients with short-lived asymptomatic arrhythmia in the outpatient settings. In contrast, in our study, we examined the triggers for heart failure hospitalizations in TICMP patients in inpatient settings. Here, arrhythmia recurrence was the main cause of heart failure exacerbation and hospitalization.

Our finding suggests that the clinical prognosis of these two groups of patients is similar. Hence, TICMP should not be regarded by clinicians as a benign disorder. We believe that implementation of the guidelines' recommendations of an early invasive strategy together with tight patient monitoring could lead to a reduction in clinical events and potentially improve prognosis in selected patients [30].

Study Limitations

This retrospective study comparing long-term outcomes of TICMP and IDCM in patients hospitalized with new onset heart failure has several limitations. First, this study contains single-center data with a small number of patients enrolled. However, our sample size is relatively large in comparison with previous studies and only a few multicenter studies included a larger study population [31,32]. Second, the follow-up clinical data were retrieved from Sheba Medical Center records only. This could lead to a possible underestimation of clinical events that patients presented with them to a different hospital. However, the majority of patients admitted to Sheba Medical Center are nearby residents that would probably be readmitted to the same medical center when experiencing a recurrence of their heart condition. Moreover, the outpatient clinic follow-up data include information about recent hospitalizations in different hospitals. By reviewing the outpatient clinic follow-up, we were able to minimize this underestimation.

Third, in our cohort, we did not find a significant difference in mortality between groups, but a larger sample size and longer follow-ups are needed to validate our result. Fourth, data on all-cause mortality were retrieved from government records. These data do not include the etiology of death. Therefore, we could not rule out differences in cardiovascular mortality between groups.

Fifth, the cohort enrolled patients from 2007 to 2017 where a more conservative treatment strategy was taken, and an ablation catheter was not considered the treatment of choice. Implantation of recent guidelines from 2020 which advocates catheter ablation to reverse LV dysfunction when TICMP is highly probable might improve the outcome of TICMP and reduce heart failure hospitalization [30].

5. Conclusions

TICMP, though at first glance appears to be a relatively benign process, has similar long-term outcomes as IDCM even following the improvement of LVEF. In fact, it portends higher rates of worsening heart failure readmissions, mostly due to arrhythmia recurrences. Further studies are needed to evaluate whether early intervention and tight rhythm monitoring can lead to a better prognosis.

Supplementary Materials: The following supporting information can be downloaded at: https://www.mdpi.com/article/10.3390/jcm12041412/s1, Table S1: History of arrhythmia and rhythm at presentation; Table S2: Devices implanted and echocardiographic parameters collected during follow-up.

Author Contributions: Conceptualization, M.K.; Formal analysis, M.K.; Data curation, A.M. and M.A.; Writing—original draft, M.K. and A.M.; Writing—review & editing, A.A. and R.B.; Supervision, M.A., E.N. and R.B. All authors have read and agreed to the published version of the manuscript.

Funding: This research received no external funding.

Institutional Review Board Statement: The study was conducted in accordance with the Declaration of Helsinki and approved by the Institutional Review Board and Ethics Committee of Haim Sheba Medical Center. Study number: 1864-14-SMC.

Informed Consent Statement: Patient consent was waived due to the retrospective nature of the study and the fact that the analyses used de-identified clinical data.

Data Availability Statement: Data are available upon request.

Conflicts of Interest: The authors declare no conflict of interest.

References

1. Huizar, J.F.; Ellenbogen, K.A.; Tan, A.Y.; Kaszala, K. Arrhythmia-Induced Cardiomyopathy: JACC State-of-the-Art Review. *J. Am. Coll. Cardiol.* **2019**, *73*, 2328–2344. [CrossRef] [PubMed]
2. Martin, C.A.; Lambiase, P.D. Pathophysiology, diagnosis and treatment of tachycardiomyopathy. *Heart* **2017**, *103*, 1543–1552. [CrossRef] [PubMed]
3. Omichi, C.; Tanaka, T.; Kakizawa, Y.; Yamada, A.; Ishii, Y.; Nagashima, H.; Kanmatsuse, K.; Endo, M. Improvement of cardiac function and neurological remodeling in a patient with tachycardia-induced cardiomyopathy after catheter ablation. *J. Cardiol.* **2009**, *54*, 134–138. [CrossRef] [PubMed]
4. Dhawan, R.; Gopinathannair, R. Arrhythmia-Induced Cardiomyopathy: Prevalent, Under-recognized, Reversible. *J. Atr. Fibrillation* **2017**, *10*, 1776. [CrossRef] [PubMed]
5. Donghua, Z.; Jian, P.; Zhongbo, X.; Feifei, Z.; Xinhui, P.; Hao, Y.; Fuqiang, L.; Yan, L.; Yong, X.; Xinfu, H.; et al. Reversal of cardiomyopathy in patients with congestive heart failure secondary to tachycardia. *J. Interv. Card. Electrophysiol.* **2013**, *36*, 27–32; discussion 32. [CrossRef]
6. Lishmanov, A.; Chockalingam, P.; Senthilkumar, A.; Chockalingam, A. Tachycardia-induced cardiomyopathy: Evaluation and therapeutic options. *Congest. Heart Fail.* **2010**, *16*, 122–126. [CrossRef]
7. Zimmermann, A.J.; Bossard, M.; Aeschbacher, S.; Schoen, T.; Voellmin, G.; Suter, Y.; Lehmann, A.; Hochgruber, T.; Pumpol, K.; Sticherling, C.; et al. Effects of sinus rhythm maintenance on left heart function after electrical cardioversion of atrial fibrillation: Implications for tachycardia-induced cardiomyopathy. *Can. J. Cardiol.* **2015**, *31*, 36–43. [CrossRef]
8. Nerheim, P.; Birger-Botkin, S.; Piracha, L.; Olshansky, B. Heart failure and sudden death in patients with tachycardia-induced cardiomyopathy and recurrent tachycardia. *Circulation* **2004**, *110*, 247–252. [CrossRef]
9. Watanabe, H.; Okamura, K.; Chinushi, M.; Furushima, H.; Tanabe, Y.; Kodama, M.; Aizawa, Y. Clinical characteristics, treatment, and outcome of tachycardia induced cardiomyopathy. *Int. Heart J.* **2008**, *49*, 39–47. [CrossRef]

10. Medi, C.; Kalman, J.M.; Haqqani, H.; Vohra, J.K.; Morton, J.B.; Sparks, P.B.; Kistler, P.M. Tachycardia-mediated cardiomyopathy secondary to focal atrial tachycardia: Long-term outcome after catheter ablation. *J. Am. Coll. Cardiol.* **2009**, *53*, 1791–1797. [CrossRef]
11. Merlo, M.; Pivetta, A.; Pinamonti, B.; Stolfo, D.; Zecchin, M.; Barbati, G.; Di Lenarda, A.; Sinagra, G. Long-term prognostic impact of therapeutic strategies in patients with idiopathic dilated cardiomyopathy: Changing mortality over the last 30 years. *Eur. J. Heart Fail.* **2014**, *16*, 317–324. [CrossRef] [PubMed]
12. Jeong, Y.H.; Choi, K.J.; Song, J.M.; Hwang, E.S.; Park, K.M.; Nam, G.B.; Kim, J.J.; Kim, Y.H. Diagnostic approach and treatment strategy in tachycardia-induced cardiomyopathy. *Clin. Cardiol.* **2008**, *31*, 172–178. [CrossRef] [PubMed]
13. McDonagh, T.A.; Metra, M.; Adamo, M.; Gardner, R.S.; Baumbach, A.; Böhm, M.; Burri, H.; Butler, J.; Čelutkienė, J.; Chioncel, O.; et al. 2021 ESC Guidelines for the diagnosis and treatment of acute and chronic heart failure: Developed by the Task Force for the diagnosis and treatment of acute and chronic heart failure of the European Society of Cardiology (ESC) With the special contribution of the Heart Failure Association (HFA) of the ESC. *Eur. Heart J.* **2021**, *42*, 3599–3726. [PubMed]
14. Jefferies, J.L.; Towbin, J.A. Dilated cardiomyopathy. *Lancet* **2010**, *375*, 752–762. [CrossRef]
15. Pinto, Y.M.; Elliott, P.M.; Arbustini, E.; Adler, Y.; Anastasakis, A.; Böhm, M.; Duboc, D.; Gimeno, J.; de Groote, P.; Imazio, M.; et al. Proposal for a revised definition of dilated cardiomyopathy, hypokinetic non-dilated cardiomyopathy, and its implications for clinical practice: A position statement of the ESC working group on myocardial and pericardial diseases. *Eur. Heart J.* **2016**, *37*, 1850–1858. [CrossRef]
16. Elliott, P.; Andersson, B.; Arbustini, E.; Bilinska, Z.; Cecchi, F.; Charron, P.; Dubourg, O.; Kuhl, U.; Maisch, B.; McKenna, W.J.; et al. Classification of the cardiomyopathies: A position statement from the European Society of Cardiology Working Group on Myocardial and Pericardial Diseases. *Eur. Heart J.* **2008**, *29*, 270–276. [CrossRef]
17. Luk, A.; Ahn, E.; Soor, G.S.; Butany, J. Dilated cardiomyopathy: A review. *J. Clin. Pathol.* **2009**, *62*, 219–225. [CrossRef]
18. Felker, G.M.; Thompson, R.E.; Hare, J.M.; Hruban, R.H.; Clemetson, D.E.; Howard, D.L.; Baughman, K.L.; Kasper, E.K. Underlying causes and long-term survival in patients with initially unexplained cardiomyopathy. *N. Engl. J. Med.* **2000**, *342*, 1077–1084. [CrossRef]
19. Ellis, E.R.; Josephson, M.E. What About Tachycardia-induced Cardiomyopathy? *Arrhythmia Electrophysiol. Rev.* **2013**, *2*, 82–90. [CrossRef]
20. Blanc, J.-J.; Fatemi, M.; Bertault, V.; Baraket, F.; Etienne, Y. Evaluation of left bundle branch block as a reversible cause of non-ischaemic dilated cardiomyopathy with severe heart failure. A new concept of left ventricular dyssynchrony-induced cardiomyopathy. *Europace* **2005**, *7*, 604–610. [CrossRef]
21. Vernooy, K.; Verbeek, X.A.; Peschar, M.; Crijns, H.J.; Arts, T.; Cornelussen, R.N.; Prinzen, F.W. Left bundle branch block induces ventricular remodelling and functional septal hypoperfusion. *Eur. Heart J.* **2005**, *26*, 91–98. [CrossRef]
22. Shamim, W.; Yousufuddin, M.; Cicoria, M.; Gibson, D.G.; Coats, A.J.; Henein, M.Y. Incremental changes in QRS duration in serial ECGs over time identify high risk elderly patients with heart failure. *Heart* **2002**, *88*, 47–51. [CrossRef] [PubMed]
23. Prinzen, F.W.; Auricchio, A.; Mullens, W.; Linde, C.; Huizar, J.F. Electrical management of heart failure: From pathophysiology to treatment. *Eur. Heart J.* **2022**, *43*, 1917–1927. [CrossRef]
24. Lund, L.H.; Benson, L.; Ståhlberg, M.; Braunschweig, F.; Edner, M.; Dahlström, U.; Linde, C. Age, prognostic impact of QRS prolongation and left bundle branch block, and utilization of cardiac resynchronization therapy: Findings from 14,713 patients in the Swedish Heart Failure Registry. *Eur. J. Heart Fail.* **2014**, *16*, 1073–1081. [CrossRef]
25. Vera, A.; Cecconi, A.; Martínez-Vives, P.; Olivera, M.J.; Hernández, S.; López-Melgar, B.; Rojas-González, A.; Díez-Villanueva, P.; Salamanca, J.; Tejelo, J.; et al. Electrocardiogram and CMR to differentiate tachycardia-induced cardiomyopathy from dilated cardiomyopathy in patients admitted for heart failure. *Heart Vessel.* **2022**, *37*, 1850–1858. [CrossRef] [PubMed]
26. DeVore, A.D.; Hellkamp, A.S.; Thomas, L.; Albert, N.M.; Butler, J.; Patterson, J.H.; Spertus, J.A.; Williams, F.B.; Shen, X.; Hernandez, A.F.; et al. The association of improvement in left ventricular ejection fraction with outcomes in patients with heart failure with reduced ejection fraction: Data from CHAMP-HF. *Eur. J. Heart Fail.* **2022**, *24*, 762–770. [CrossRef] [PubMed]
27. Dries, D.L.; Exner, D.V.; Gersh, B.J.; Domanski, M.J.; Waclawiw, M.A.; Stevenson, L.W. Atrial fibrillation is associated with an increased risk for mortality and heart failure progression in patients with asymptomatic and symptomatic left ventricular systolic dysfunction: A retrospective analysis of the SOLVD trials. Studies of Left Ventricular Dysfunction. *J. Am. Coll. Cardiol.* **1998**, *32*, 695–703.
28. Meltzer, R.S.; Visser, C.A.; Fuster, V. Intracardiac thrombi and systemic embolization. *Ann. Intern. Med.* **1986**, *104*, 689–698. [CrossRef]
29. Ahmad, A.; Mar, P.L.; Olshansky, B.; Horbal, P.; Tsai, C.; Patel, H.; Hussein, A.; Dickey, S.; Dhawan, R.; Murray, A.; et al. Echocardiographic changes and heart failure hospitalizations following rhythm control for arrhythmia-induced cardiomyopathy: Results from a multicenter, retrospective study. *J. Interv. Card. Electrophysiol.* **2022**. [CrossRef]
30. Hindricks, G.; Potpara, T.; Dagres, N.; Arbelo, E.; Bax, J.J.; Blomström-Lundqvist, C.; Boriani, G.; Castella, M.; Dan, G.-A.; Dilaveri, P.; et al. 2020 ESC Guidelines for the diagnosis and management of atrial fibrillation developed in collaboration with the European Association for Cardio-Thoracic Surgery (EACTS): The Task Force for the diagnosis and management of atrial fibrillation of the European Society of Cardiology (ESC) Developed with the special contribution of the European Heart Rhythm Association (EHRA) of the ESC. *Eur. Heart J.* **2020**, *42*, 373–498.

31. Montero, S.; Ferrero-Gregori, A.; Cinca, J.; Guerra, J.M. Long-term Outcome of Patients with Tachycardia-induced Cardiomyopathy After Recovery of Left Ventricular Function. *Rev. Esp. Cardiol.* **2018**, *71*, 681–683. [CrossRef] [PubMed]
32. Zhang, H.; Lu, D.; Tang, X. Radiofrequency catheter ablation improves long-term prognosis and cardiac function of the patients with tachyarrhythmia-induced cardiomyopathy. *Int. J. Clin. Pr.* **2021**, *75*, e14007. [CrossRef] [PubMed]

Disclaimer/Publisher's Note: The statements, opinions and data contained in all publications are solely those of the individual author(s) and contributor(s) and not of MDPI and/or the editor(s). MDPI and/or the editor(s) disclaim responsibility for any injury to people or property resulting from any ideas, methods, instructions or products referred to in the content.

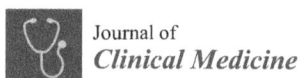 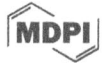

Article

A Referral Center Experience with Cerebral Protection Devices: Challenging Cardiac Thrombus in the EP Lab

Jan Berg [1,2,*], Alberto Preda [1], Nicolai Fierro [1], Alessandra Marzi [1], Andrea Radinovic [1], Paolo Della Bella [1] and Patrizio Mazzone [1]

1. Division of Arrhythmology, San Raffaele Hospital, 20132 Milan, Italy
2. Division of Cardiology, Cantonal Hospital of Aarau, 5001 Aarau, Switzerland
* Correspondence: jan.berg@ksa.ch

Abstract: BACKGROUND: Cerebral protection devices (CPD) are designed to prevent cardioembolic stroke and most evidence that exists relates to TAVR procedures. There are missing data on the benefits of CPD in patients that are considered high risk for stroke undergoing cardiac procedures like left atrial appendage (LAA) closure or catheter ablation of ventricular tachycardia (VT) when cardiac thrombus is present. PURPOSE: This work aimed to examine the feasibility and safety of the routine use of CPD in patients with cardiac thrombus undergoing interventions in the electrophysiology (EP) lab of a large referral center. METHODS: The CPD was placed under fluoroscopic guidance in all procedures in the beginning of the intervention. Two different CPDs were used according to the physician's discretion: (1) a capture device consisting of two filters for the brachiocephalic and left common carotid arteries placed over a 6F sheath from a radial artery; or (2) a deflection device covering all three supra-aortic vessels placed over an 8F femoral sheath. Retrospective periprocedural and safety data were obtained from procedural reports and discharge letters. Long-term safety data were obtained by clinical follow-up in our institution and telephone consultations. RESULTS: We identified 30 consecutive patients in our EP lab who underwent interventions (21 LAA closure, 9 VT ablation) with placement of a CPD due to cardiac thrombus. Mean age was 70 ± 10 years and 73% were male, while mean LVEF was 40 ± 14%. The location of the cardiac thrombus was the LAA in all 21 patients (100%) undergoing LAA-closure, whereas, in the 9 patients undergoing VT ablation, thrombus was present in the LAA in 5 cases (56%), left ventricle (n = 3, 33%) and aortic arch (n = 1, 11%). The capture device was used in 19 out of 30 (63%) and the deflection device in 11 out of 30 cases (37%). There were no periprocedural strokes or transitory ischemic attacks (TIA). CPD-related complications comprised the vascular access and were as follows: two cases of pseudoaneurysm of the femoral artery not requiring surgery (7%), 1 hematoma at the arterial puncture site (3%) and 1 venous thrombosis (3%) resolved by warfarin. At long-term follow-up, 1 TIA and 2 non-cardiovascular deaths occurred, with a mean follow-up time of 660 days. CONCLUSIONS: Placement of a cerebral protection device prior to LAA closure or VT ablation in patients with cardiac thrombus proved feasible, but possible vascular complications needed to be taken into account. A benefit in periprocedural stroke prevention for these interventions seemed plausible but has yet to be proven in larger and randomized trials.

Keywords: left atrial appendage closure; catheter ablation; stroke; cerebral protection

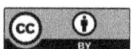

1. Introduction

Stroke following electrophysiologic (EP) interventions of the heart is a serious complication. Periprocedural stroke risk is estimated between 0.1–0.9% in patients undergoing catheter ablation of atrial fibrillation [1–4], between 0.8–1.8% in patients undergoing ablation of ventricular tachycardia (VT) [4–6] and 0.7–1.1% in patients undergoing endocardial appendage closure [7,8]. Therefore, it is crucial to reduce stroke risk in patients that are considered high risk of periprocedural stroke. However, strategies to avoid periprocedural stroke are not well established in the general EP lab. Recently, cerebral protection devices (CPD) have become commercially available; the two most frequently used systems are the Sentinel © (Boston Scientific, Marlborough, MA, USA) and the Triguard © system (Keystone Heart, Caesarea, Israel). These two CPD differ in deployment and arrangement, and both systems have been widely studied in transcatheter aortic valve replacement (TAVR) procedures [9–15].

However, there are insufficient data about the benefits of CPD in EP procedures. To our knowledge, there have been two small studies with CPD in patients undergoing ablation of ventricular tachycardia. The first study reported feasibility and safety in a series of 11 patients with ischemic heart disease undergoing VT ablation [16] using the Sentinel© CPD device. The authors reported detection of debris in the device after the procedure in all patients, highlighting the plausibility of using CPDs in patients undergoing procedures with elevated stroke risk. In a second study, our group reported on the feasibility and safety of using the Sentinel and Triguard CPD in 7 patients undergoing ablation of ventricular tachycardia [17]. Recently, the feasibility of left atrial appendage (LAA) closure in presence of a cardiac thrombus was reported for the Sentinel [18,19] and the Triguard device [20].

The aim of this study was to provide data on the feasibility of using the two most common CPD in patients with cardiac thrombus undergoing cardiac interventions in the EP lab of a large tertiary center—and to report periprocedural and long-term outcomes in this selected group.

2. Materials and Methods

We conducted a single-center retrospective and observational study, including all patients undergoing procedures with deployment of a CPD, in the EP labs of the Arrhythmology Department at San Raffaele Hospital, Milan, Italy between June 2016 and April 2022. A total of 32 consecutive patients were identified; 2 had to be excluded because of insufficient data. The study was conducted according to institutional guidelines and legal requirements and complied with the Declaration of Helsinki.

2.1. Clinical and Echocardiographic Data

Baseline clinical data were retrospectively collected by clinical chart review. All patients underwent baseline transthoracic echocardiography (TTE). Transoesophageal echocardiography (TOE) was performed in all patients with planned endocardial LAA closure. During TOE, thrombotic material was classified as either sludge or manifest thrombus. TTE and TOE were conducted with a Vivid E95 (GE healthcare, USA) and a M5Sc probe for TTE and 6VT-D probe for TOE.

2.2. Procedures

All procedures were conducted in general anesthesia. The CPD was placed under fluoroscopic guidance in all procedures in the beginning of the procedure, before a transseptal puncture. There was one experienced operator for LAA closure and one experienced operator for VT ablation, respectively, who were responsible for the main procedure and placement of the protection device. Both operators were assisted by at least one experienced electrophysiologist or fellow during the procedure.

2.2.1. Sentinel Device

The Sentinel CPD is a capture device consisting of two polyurethane filters with 140-μm-diameter pores designed to capture thrombotic material. It is inserted from a radial or brachial artery over a 6F delivery catheter with a deflectable distal tip. The proximal filter is placed in the brachiocephalic trunk, the distal filter is placed in the left common carotid artery (Figure 1; online Supplemental Video S1). Before device placement, the aortic branches are visualized by contrast angiography over a pigtail catheter which is placed in the ascending aorta.

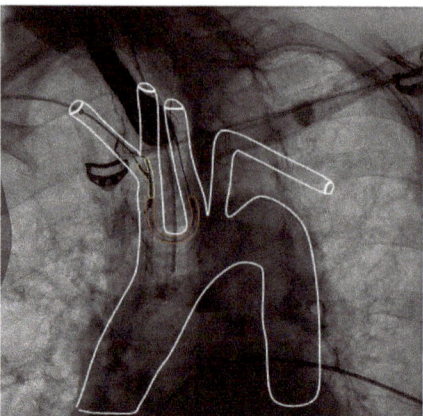

Figure 1. The Sentinel device in standard position, covering the brachiocephalic and left common carotid artery. Anteroposterior view. Aortic arch and supraaortic vessels are depicted in white, the device is depicted in yellow for better visibility.

2.2.2. Triguard 3 Device

The Triguard 3 CPD is a deflection device which covers all three supra-aortic vessels (brachiocephalic, left common carotid and left subclavian arteries, Figure 2; online Supplemental Video S2) with a polymeric mesh, with a pore size of 115 × 145 μm. It is placed over an 8F delivery catheter from a femoral artery and designed to self-position in the aortic arch.

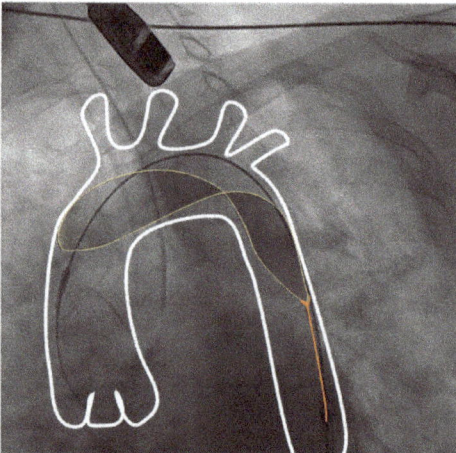

Figure 2. Triguard device in standard position covering the supra-aortic vessels. Anteroposterior view. Aortic arch and supraaortic vessels are depicted in white, the device is depicted in yellow for better visibility.

2.2.3. LAA Closure Procedure

LAA closure was conducted in general anesthesia using no-touch implantation technique in order to avoid dislodgement of thrombotic material, as previously described by our group [18]. A single puncture of the fossa ovalis was performed from the infero-posterior site for optimal alignment with the LAA. After transseptal puncture, intravenous heparin was administered with a goal of 300 s of activated clotting time (ACT). The evaluation of the LAA anatomy to select the correct device size was performed with TOE in all cases and, only in the case of suboptimal imaging, a small dose of contrast agent was manually injected with a pigtail catheter near the LAA ostium without advancing it deeply into the LAA. The device was unsheathed and later completely deployed under TOE and fluoroscopic monitoring. Device stability was assessed with the tug test, and the result was confirmed by angiography. Small thrombotic debris were eventually captured in the CPD at the end of the procedure. Finally, the correct positioning and the absence of significant peri-device leaks were confirmed by angiography and 2D/3D TOE. After the procedure, hemostasis was reached through removal of the sheath and subsequent manual compression of the venous and arterial access sites, when the ACT was less than 180 s.

2.2.4. VT Ablation Procedure

VT ablations were performed under general anesthesia using the standard approach in our institution, as published previously [21]. Programmed electrical stimulation was utilized to induce the VT. For the antegrade approach, venous access was obtained via the right femoral vein and a single transseptal puncture was performed under fluoroscopic guidance. For the retrograde approach, an 8F sheath was advanced into the descending aorta via the right femoral artery. An ACT level of 300 s was aimed during the procedure. LV mapping was conducted utilizing either the CARTO 3 (Biosense Webster, Inc.) or the ENSITE X electroanatomical mapping system (Abbott, MN, USA). The geometry of the chamber was reconstructed in sinus rhythm with the ablation catheter and then refined with a high density multipolar mapping catheter. Scar zones and local late potentials were mapped. Additional epicardial mapping and ablation was performed in patients with an ECG morphology or a substrate suggestive of an epicardial origin. If a hemodynamically stable VT could be induced, the critical isthmus of the VT was mapped with the multipolar catheter and ablated. For hemodynamically unstable VT, pace mapping was performed at different sites within the low-voltage area during sinus rhythm to identify the VT exit and potential critical isthmus. Radiofrequency current was delivered with a maximum power of 50W. The procedural end point was the elimination of late potentials and the non-inducibility of any sustained VT via programmed electrical stimulation.

2.3. Periprocedural Events and Follow-Up

Information about periprocedural outcomes, including all procedure and device-related adverse events (<7 days), were taken from patient charts and electronic patient files. Complications were divided into two categories: (1) related to the CPD or (2) not related to the CPD.

Additional long-term follow-up was conducted by follow-up visits in our outpatient clinic or, if not available, by telephone interviews with the patient. Main focus of long-term follow-up was to assess safety of our approach and possible complications. Routine clinical follow-up visits included a clinical anamnesis, ECG and a medical examination in our outpatient clinic. Patients, after LAA closure, underwent additional TOE after 3 to 6 months in our clinic or at the referring center. Follow-up of patients after VT ablation was scheduled according to the physician's discretion. Telephone interviews were conducted retrospectively in patients where clinical follow-up was not available and aimed for events like vascular complications or TIA/stroke.

2.4. Statistical Analysis

Continuous variables are expressed as mean ± standard deviation. Categorical variables are expressed as numbers and percentage. The authors decided to report descriptive data, rather than using statistical tests, in this selected and heterogenous group, with low event rates and low patient numbers. All authors had full access to all the data in the study and have taken responsibility for its integrity and that of the data analysis.

3. Results
3.1. Clinical Characteristics

Thirty consecutive patients were included in the final analysis. Baseline characteristics are summarized in Table 1. Mean age in the entire patient cohort was 70.2 ± 10.2 (range 37–87) years and 22 out of 30 patients (73%) were male. Mean CHA2DS2VASC-score was 3.2 ± 1.4 and mean HASBLED score 2.1 ± 0.8. Mean left ventricular ejection fraction was 40.2 ± 13.6. Most patients had ischemic cardiomyopathy (n = 10, 33%) as the underlying disease. Five patients (17%) had dilated cardiomyopathy, 3 patients (10%) tachycardiomyopathy, 2 primary valvular cardiomyopathy (7%), 1 rheumatic heart disease (3%) and 1 hypertrophic cardiomyopathy (3%). Additionally, 12 patients (40%) had undergone cardiac surgery before, with valvular surgery (n = 6; 20%) being the most prevalent, followed by coronary artery bypass grafting (n = 4; 13%), left ventricular aneurysmectomy (n = 1; 3%) and myectomy (n = 1; 3%). Finally, 2 patients (7%) were pacemaker carriers, and 12 patients (40%) were carriers of an implantable cardioverter-defibrillator.

Table 1. Baseline characteristics.

Variable	Total	LAA Closure	VT Ablation
No. Patients, n	30	21	9
Age, mean ± SD	70.2 ± 10.2	70.1 ± 11	70.6 ± 7.7
Female gender	8 (27%)	8 (31%)	--
Comorbidities			
Hypertension	16 (53%)	12 (57%)	4 (44%)
Dyslipidemia	10 (33%)	8 (38%)	2 (22%)
Diabetes Mellitus	2 (7%)	2 (10%)	--
Coronary artery disease	10 (33%)	6 (29%)	4 (44%)
Atrial Fibrillation, n (%)	28 (93%)	21 (100%)	7 (78%)
Paroxysmal	1 (3%)	--	1 (11%)
Persistent	16 (53%)	13 (62%)	3 (33%)
Long-standing persistent	2 (7%)	2 (10%)	--
Permanent	9 (30%)	6 (29%)	3 (33%)
Congestive Heart Failure	21 (70%)	12 (57%)	9 (100%)
PM	2 (7%)	2 (10%)	--
ICD	12 (40%)	3 (14%)	9 (100%)
Stroke or TIA history	2 (7%)	2 (10%)	--
Systemic arterial embolism	1 (3%)	1 (5%)	--
Bleeding predisposition	12 (40%)	10 (48%)	2 (22%)
Intracranial Hemorrhage	6 (20%)	5 (24%)	1 (11%)
GI bleeding	2 (6%)	2 (10%)	--
Diffuse bleeding with anemia	1 (3%)	1 (5%)	--
Teleangiectasia in Rendu-Osler-Weber disease	1 (3%)	1 (5%)	--
Intraretinal bleeding	1 (3%)	1 (5%)	--
Hemophilia A	1 (3%)	--	1 (11%)
Previous cardiac surgery	12 (40%)	7 (33%)	5 (56%)
Coronary bypass surgery	4 (13%)	3 (10%)	1 (11%)
Valvular surgery	6 (20%)	4 (13%)	2 (22%)
Myectomy	1 (3%)	--	1 (11%)
LV aneurysmectomy	1 (3%)	--	1 (11%)
Cardiomyopathies, n (%)	22 (73%)	13 (62%)	9 (100%)
Ischemic cardiomyopathy	10 (33%)	6 (29%)	4 (44%)
Dilated cardiomyopathy	5 (17%)	2 (10%)	3 (33%)
Primary valvular cardiomyopathy	2 (7%)	2 (10%)	--

Table 1. Cont.

Variable	Total	LAA Closure	VT Ablation
Hypertrophic cardiomyopathy	1 (3%)	--	1 (11%)
Tachycardiomyopathy	3 (10%)	3 (14%)	--
Rheumatic heart disease	1 (3%)	--	1 (11%)
Risk scores			
CHA2DS2-VASc, mean ± SD	3.2 ± 1.4	3.2 ± 1.4	3.1 ± 1.4
HASBLED, mean ± SD	2.1 ± 0.8	2.1 ± 0.9	2.3 ± 0.7
Antithrombotic treatment	26 (84%)	17 (81%)	9 (100%)
Low dose Aspirin	4 (13%)	2 (10%)	2 (22%)
DOAC	9 (30%)	8 (38%)	1 (11%)
VKA	13 (43%)	7 (33%)	6 (67%)
Echo characteristics			
LVEF, mean ± SD %	40.2 ± 13.6	45.8 ± 10.1	29.6 ± 13.1
LAA thrombus or significant sludge before procedure	26 (87%)	21 (100%)	5 (56%)
LV thrombus or significant sludge before procedure	3 (10%)	--	3 (33%)
mobile thrombus in aortic arch	1 (3%)	--	1 (11%)

Abbreviations: CAD, coronary artery disease; DOAC, direct oral anticoagulant; GI, gastro intestinal; ICD, internal cardioverter-defibrillator defibrillator; LAA, left atrial appendage;; LV, left ventricle; LVEF, Left Ventricular Ejection Fraction; PM, pacemaker; SD, standard deviation; TIA: transient ischemic attack; VKA, vitamin K antagonists. Congestive Heart Failure = EF < 50%.

In total, 21 patients (70%) underwent LAA closure, whereas 13 of those (62%) received an Amplatzer Amulet and 8 (38%) received a Watchman FLX device. Among those 21 patients who underwent LAA closure, a manifest thrombus in the LAA was found in 16 cases (76%), whereas severe sludge in LAA was found in 5 cases (24%). The most common indication for LAA closure was persistent thrombus despite anticoagulation in 13 cases (62%), a strategy previously described by our group [18] and in a meta-analysis [20]. Other indications were: inability to take oral anticoagulation because of intracranial bleeding in 5 (24%), gastrointestinal bleeding in 2 (10%) and diffuse bleeding with anemia in 1 (5%). Atrial fibrillation (AF) was present in all patients undergoing LAA closure (21 out of 21 patients). AF pattern was persistent in 13 (62%), long-standing persistent in 2 (10%) and permanent in 6 patients (29%).

Nine patients (30%) underwent VT ablation. Among those patients, a manifest thrombus in the LAA was found in 5 (56%), a left ventricular thrombus was found in 2 (22%), severe spontaneous echo contrast in the left ventricle in 1 (11%) and mobile thrombotic material in the aortic arch in 1 (11%), prior to the intervention as a reason for using a CPD. AF was present in 7 patients (78%) undergoing VT ablation (persistent n = 3, permanent n = 3, paroxysmal n = 1).

3.2. Procedural Data

Placement of the CPD was feasible in all patients; the Sentinel device was used in 19 out of 30 (63%) and the Triguard 3 device in 11 out of 30 cases (37%). Mean procedure time including placement of the CPD was 103 ± 25 min for LAA closure and 246 ± 29 min for VT ablation. Mean hospitalization time was 2.9 ± 2.2 days in LAA closure and 14.3 ± 12.2 days for VT ablation. The mean number of vascular access sheaths was 3.8 ± 0.7 per procedure.

3.3. Periprocedural Complications

Data about periprocedural complications until discharge were available for all patients.
Periprocedural complications were noted in 3 out of 21 patients undergoing LAAC (14%). Those were (1) hematoma of the right arm at the arterial puncture site with swollen extremity in 1 patient which resolved spontaneously, (2) thrombosis of the right communal

femoral vein in 1 patient which was later resolved by warfarin, and (3) pseudoaneurysm of the right femoral artery which did not require surgery. All 3 complications were categorized as possibly related to the placement of the CPD.

Periprocedural complications occurred in 4 out of 9 patients (44%) undergoing VT ablation with a CPD. One patient died in-hospital after VT ablation, not related to placement of the CPD. Other complications were cardiogenic shock with insertion of an intra-aortic balloon pump in 2 patients with VT ablation, also not related to the CPD. A pseudoaneurysm of the left superficial femoral artery not requiring surgery was noted in 1 patient, which was categorized as possibly related to the CPD.

In summary, there were 4 complications related to the CPD in 30 patients (13%). All complications comprised the vascular access site and none of the complications required surgery (Table 2).

Table 2. CPD-related complications.

LAA Closure with Sentinel	LAA Closure with Triguard	VT Ablation with Sentinel	VT Ablation with Triguard
14	7	5	4
Hematoma = 1 Venous thrombosis = 1	Arterial pseudoaneurysm = 1	--	Arterial pseudoaneurysm = 1

3.4. Follow-Up

Long-term follow-up data were available for 26 out of 30 patients (87%) and mean follow-up time was 660 days. At long-term follow-up 1 TIA and 2 non-cardiovascular deaths (1 death because of gastric cancer 575 days after LAA closure, 1 death because of pneumonia 587 days after LAA closure) were noted during long-term follow-up.

4. Discussion

4.1. Main Study Findings

The main findings of this study were the following: (1) application of the Sentinel and Triguard CPD was feasible in all patients undergoing LAA closure and VT ablation. (2) Placement of these two different devices was safe, with vascular complications that did not require surgery as the only complications in our cohort (n = 4, 13%). (3) There were no instances of periprocedural TIA or stroke despite the presence of cardiac thrombus in all patients. Finally, long-term follow-up confirmed safety of our approach in this patient cohort at high risk for stroke.

4.2. Comparison with Other Studies

To our knowledge, this was the largest study to report on outcomes of patients undergoing cerebral embolic protection with two different devices in a general EP lab.

Very recently, the randomized protected TAVR trial did not find significant differences in stroke incidence after TAVR in patients with a Sentinel device during TAVR [22]. There was a stroke incidence of 2.3% in the CPD group and a lower than expected 2.9% stroke incidence in the control group. However, in the subgroup analysis, the authors found a higher proportion of disabling strokes in the group without CPD. This finding was hypothesis-generating, but it raised the question of whether embolic protection could be more beneficial in patients at highest risk for stroke, rather than in the general TAVR population. Given the large number needed to treat, of 125 patients in the protected TAVR trial, to avoid one disabling stroke, one could argue that patient selection is critical to gain any benefit in stroke protection. In our study, patients were considered high risk for development of stroke because cardiac thrombus was already present.

Prior studies with single devices, mostly the Sentinel device, have been published in LAA closure and VT ablation. Bocuzzi et al. [19] published data comprising 28 patients from 8 centers with AF and LAA thrombus undergoing LAA closure and cerebral protection with the Sentinel device. They found no strokes and no complications at the access site. A systematic review by Sharma et al. identified 58 patients with LAA thrombus who underwent LAA closure. Of those, 17 received cerebral protection with different devices. No strokes were reported, but vascular complications were not assessed. Heeger et al. [16] found that cerebral protection with the Sentinel device was feasible and safe in a series of 11 patients undergoing VT ablation. Importantly, VT ablation was associated with embolization of embolic debris, found in the device filter in all patients after VT ablation. The authors reported no strokes, in line with our findings. To our knowledge, the only case where a Triguard device was used for VT ablation was published by our own group. In the initial experience by Zachariah et al. [17] with 7 patients undergoing VT ablation, Triguard was used in 1 patient and Sentinel was used in 6 patients. Placement of all devices was feasible and there were no complications.

In summary, our findings were in line with previous studies in terms of feasibility and safety for the Sentinel and Triguard devices in LAA closure and VT ablation. In contrast to previous studies, we reported on complications at the access site, which need to be balanced against the possible benefits in stroke prevention.

4.3. Technical Aspects

The Sentinel CPD does not protect the left vertebral and subclavian arteries. Additionally, it requires contrast angiography of the aortic branches prior to placement and correct placement of the device requires a learning curve in our experience.

The Triguard 3 device, which covers all supra-aortic vessels with a single filter, requires less experience, in our opinion. Moreover, in our experience, contrast angiography was not always mandatory, leading to the possibility of avoiding exposition with contrast agent when necessary, as in cases with renal failure or allergy against iodine contrast agent. However, the access sheath is larger (8F femoral artery sheath in Triguard 3 versus 6F radial artery sheath in Sentinel).

We reported a relatively high number of vascular complications (4 out of 30 patients, 13%) in our cohort. Of these, 1 was a hematoma, 2 were pseudoaneurysms of the femoral artery not requiring surgery and one was a venous thrombosis which was later resolved by warfarin. Of note, these patients required a high number of sheaths (mean 3.8 sheaths per procedure) for their venous and arterial accesses, respectively. These findings highlighted the importance of a standardized protocol for venous and arterial puncture and careful consideration of the necessity for each vascular access.

4.4. Clinical Implications

Our findings showed that placement of a cerebral protection prior to LAA closure or VT ablation in patients with cardiac thrombus was feasible. However, vascular complications could occur. The availability of two different cerebral protection devices in the EP lab offers the possibility to treat patients at high risk for stroke undergoing LAA closure and VT ablation. In our opinion, the mere possibility of safely performing an LAA closure procedure in the presence of an intracardiac thrombus is a very important aspect. The possibility of treating VT by catheter ablation in the presence of an intraventricular thrombus, or protecting against atrial embolization, in case of DC cardioversion of untolerated VT, is also very important, since it opens the possibility of safely performing potentially lifesaving procedures without adding embolic risk. The results of our single-center experience may encourage clinicians to consider cerebral protection, based on a case-to-case decision, while this approach remains unestablished in international guidelines.

4.5. Limitations

We did not examine the incidence of silent new cerebral embolic lesions (CEL) after intervention, since routine cMRI procedures were not performed in clinically asymptomatic patients. A previous report detected up to 32% asymptomatic CEL after Watchman implantation [23], but incidence in our selected group of high-risk patients remains speculative.

Recent studies have shown frequent discovery of thrombotic debris in CPD [16], but we were unable to provide any data regarding this, as it was not systematically reported in our patient cohort.

5. Conclusions

Placement of a cerebral embolic protection device prior to LAA closure or VT ablation in patients with cardiac thrombus was feasible, but possible vascular complications needed to be taken into account. A benefit in periprocedural stroke prevention for these interventions seems plausible, but has yet to be proven in larger and randomized trials.

Supplementary Materials: The following supporting information can be downloaded at: https://www.mdpi.com/article/10.3390/jcm12041549/s1.

Author Contributions: Conceptualization, J.B.; Investigation, N.F. and A.M.; Writing—original draft, J.B.; Writing—review & editing, A.M., A.R., P.D.B. and P.M.; Visualization, A.P.; Supervision, A.R. and P.M. All authors have read and agreed to the published version of the manuscript.

Funding: This research received no external funding.

Institutional Review Board Statement: Data was recorded in a dedicated database in compliance with the ethic committee of our centre (Institutional Ethics Committee of San Raffaele Hospital, LAAO projects). The study was conducted according to institutional guidelines and legal requirements and complied with the Declaration of Helsinki.

Informed Consent Statement: Informed consent was obtained from all subjects involved in the study.

Data Availability Statement: The data in this study are available on request from the corresponding author.

Acknowledgments: The authors would like to thank our technician Davide Maccagni for helping with the images.

Conflicts of Interest: The authors declare no conflict of interest.

References

1. Patel, D.; Bailey, S.M.; Furlan, A.J.; Ching, M.; Zachaib, J.; Di Biase, L.; Mohanty, P.; Horton, R.P.; Burkhardt, J.D.; Sanchez, J.E.; et al. Long-Term Functional and Neurocognitive Recovery in Patients Who Had an Acute Cerebrovascular Event Secondary to Catheter Ablation for Atrial Fibrillation. *J. Cardiovasc. Electrophysiol.* **2010**, *21*, 412–417. [CrossRef]
2. Cappato, R.; Calkins, H.; Chen, S.-A.; Davies, W.; Iesaka, Y.; Kalman, J.; Kim, Y.-H.; Klein, G.; Natale, A.; Packer, D.; et al. Updated Worldwide Survey on the Methods, Efficacy, and Safety of Catheter Ablation for Human Atrial Fibrillation. *Circ. Arrhythm. Electrophysiol.* **2010**, *3*, 32–38. [CrossRef] [PubMed]
3. Santangeli, P.; Di Biase, L.; Horton, R.; Burkhardt, J.D.; Sanchez, J.; Al-Ahmad, A.; Hongo, R.; Beheiry, S.; Bai, R.; Mohanty, P.; et al. Ablation of atrial fibrillation under therapeutic warfarin reduces periprocedural complications evidence from a meta-analysis. *Circ. Arrhythm. Electrophysiol.* **2012**, *5*, 302–311. [CrossRef] [PubMed]
4. Bohnen, M.; Stevenson, W.G.; Tedrow, U.B.; Michaud, G.F.; John, R.M.; Epstein, L.M.; Albert, C.M.; Koplan, B.A. Incidence and predictors of major complications from contemporary catheter ablation to treat cardiac arrhythmias. *Heart Rhythm.* **2011**, *8*, 1661–1666. [CrossRef] [PubMed]
5. Whitman, I.R.; Gladstone, R.A.; Badhwar, N.; Hsia, H.H.; Lee, B.K.; Josephson, S.A.; Meisel, K.M.; Dillon, W.P., Jr.; Hess, C.P.; Gerstenfeld, E.P.; et al. Brain Emboli after Left Ventricular Endocardial Ablation. *Circulation* **2017**, *135*, 867–877. [CrossRef] [PubMed]
6. Kuck, K.-H.; Schaumann, A.; Eckardt, L.; Willems, S.; Ventura, R.; Delacrétaz, E.; Pitschner, H.-F.; Kautzner, J.; Schumacher, B.; Hansen, P.S. Catheter ablation of stable ventricular tachycardia before defibrillator implantation in patients with coronary heart disease (VTACH): A multicentre randomised controlled trial. *Lancet* **2010**, *375*, 31–40. [CrossRef]
7. Holmes, D.R.; Kar, S.; Price, M.J.; Whisenant, B.; Sievert, H.; Doshi, S.K.; Huber, K.; Reddy, V.Y. Prospective Randomized Evaluation of the Watchman Left Atrial Appendage Closure Device in Patients with Atrial Fibrillation Versus Long-Term Warfarin Therapy: The PREVAIL Trial. *J. Am. Coll. Cardiol.* **2014**, *64*, 1–12. [CrossRef]
8. Reddy, V.Y.; Sievert, H.; Halperin, J.; Doshi, S.K.; Buchbinder, M.; Neuzil, P.; Huber, K.; Whisenant, B.; Kar, S.; Swarup, V.; et al. Percutaneous Left Atrial Appendage Closure vs Warfarin for Atrial Fibrillation A Randomized Clinical Trial Supplemental content at jama.com Original Investigation. *JAMA* **2014**, *312*, 1988–1998. [CrossRef]

9. Kapadia, S.R.; Kodali, S.; Makkar, R.; Mehran, R.; Lazar, R.M.; Zivadinov, R.; Dwyer, M.G.; Jilaihawi, H.; Virmani, R.; Anwaruddin, S.; et al. Protection Against Cerebral Embolism During Transcatheter Aortic Valve Replacement. *J. Am. Coll. Cardiol.* **2017**, *69*, 367–377. [CrossRef]
10. Haussig, S.; Mangner, N.; Dwyer, M.G.; Lehmkuhl, L.; Lücke, C.; Woitek, F.; Holzhey, D.M.; Mohr, F.W.; Gutberlet, M.; Zivadinov, R.; et al. Effect of a cerebral protection device on brain lesions following transcatheter aortic valve implantation in patients with severe aortic stenosis: The CLEAN-TAVI randomized clinical trial. *JAMA—J. Am. Med. Assoc.* **2016**, *316*, 592–601. [CrossRef]
11. Seeger, J.; Gonska, B.; Otto, M.; Rottbauer, W.; Wöhrle, J. Cerebral Embolic Protection during Transcatheter Aortic Valve Replacement Significantly Reduces Death and Stroke Compared with Unprotected Procedures. *JACC Cardiovasc. Interv.* **2017**, *10*, 2297–2303. [CrossRef] [PubMed]
12. Van Mieghem, N.M.; van Gils, L.; Ahmad, H.; van Kesteren, F.; van der Werf, H.W.; Brueren, G.; Storm, M.; Lenzen, M.; Daemen, J.; van den Heuvel, A.F.M.; et al. Filter-based cerebral embolic protection with transcatheter aortic valve implantation: The randomised MISTRAL-C trial. *EuroIntervention* **2016**, *12*, 499–507. [CrossRef] [PubMed]
13. Nazif, T.M.; Moses, J.; Sharma, R.; Dhoble, A.; Rovin, J.; Brown, D.; Horwitz, P.; Makkar, R.; Stoler, R.; Forrest, J.; et al. Randomized Evaluation of TriGuard 3 Cerebral Embolic Protection After Transcatheter Aortic Valve Replacement: Reflect II. *JACC Cardiovasc. Interv.* **2021**, *14*, 515–527. [CrossRef] [PubMed]
14. Baumbach, A.; Mullen, M.; Brickman, A.M.; Aggarwal, S.K.; Pietras, C.G.; Forrest, J.K.; Hildick-Smith, D.; Meller, S.M.; Gambone, L.; den Heijer, P.; et al. Safety and performance of a novel embolic deflection device in patients undergoing transcatheter aortic valve replacement: Results from the DEFLECT I study. *EuroIntervention* **2015**, *11*, 75–84. [CrossRef]
15. Lansky, A.J.; Schofer, J.; Tchetche, D.; Stella, P.; Pietras, C.G.; Parise, H.; Abrams, K.; Forrest, J.K.; Cleman, M.; Reinöhl, J.; et al. A prospective randomized evaluation of the Triguardtm HDH embolic Deflection device during transcatheter aortic valve implantation: Results from the DEFLECT III trial. *Eur. Heart J.* **2015**, *36*, 2070–2078. [CrossRef]
16. Heeger, C.; Metzner, A.; Schlüter, M.; Rillig, A.; Mathew, S.; Tilz, R.R.; Wohlmuth, P.; Romero, M.E.; Virmani, R.; Fink, T.; et al. Cerebral Protection during Catheter Ablation of Ventricular Tachycardia in Patients with Ischemic Heart Disease. *J. Am. Heart Assoc.* **2018**, *7*, e009005. [CrossRef]
17. Zachariah, D.; Limite, L.R.; Mazzone, P.; Marzi, A.; Radinovic, A.; Baratto, F.; Italia, L.; Ancona, F.; Paglino, G.; Della Bella, P. Use of Cerebral Protection Device in Patients Undergoing Ventricular Tachycardia Catheter Ablation. *JACC Clin. Electrophysiol.* **2022**, *8*, 528–530. [CrossRef]
18. Limite, L.R.; Radinovic, A.; Cianfanelli, L.; Altizio, S.; Peretto, G.; Frontera, A.; D'Angelo, G.; Baratto, F.; Marzi, A.; Ancona, F.; et al. Outcome of left atrial appendage closure using cerebral protection system for thrombosis: No patient left behind. *Pacing Clin. Electrophysiol.* **2022**, *45*, 23–34. [CrossRef]
19. Boccuzzi, G.G.; Montabone, A.; D'Ascenzo, F.; Colombo, F.; Ugo, F.; Muraglia, S.; De Backer, O.; Nombela-Franco, L.; Meincke, F.; Mazzone, P. Cerebral protection in left atrial appendage closure in the presence of appendage thrombosis. *Catheter. Cardiovasc. Interv.* **2021**, *97*, 511–515. [CrossRef]
20. Sharma, S.P.; Cheng, J.; Turagam, M.K.; Gopinathannair, R.; Horton, R.; Lam, Y.-Y.; Tarantini, G.; D'Amico, G.; Freixa Rofastes, X.; Lange, M.; et al. Feasibility of Left Atrial Appendage Occlusion in Left Atrial Appendage Thrombus: A Systematic Review. *JACC Clin Electrophysiol.* **2020**, *6*, 414–424. [CrossRef]
21. Zachariah, D.; Nakajima, K.; Limite, L.R.; Zweiker, D.; Spartalis, M.; Zirolia, D.; Musto, M.; D'Angelo, G.; Paglino, G.; Baratto, F.; et al. Significance of Abnormal and Late Ventricular Signatures in Ventricular Tachycardia Ablation of Ischaemic and Non-Ischaemic Cardiomyopathies. *Heart Rhythm.* **2022**, *19*, P2075–P2083. Available online: https://linkinghub.elsevier.com/retrieve/pii/S1547527122022937 (accessed on 29 December 2022). [CrossRef] [PubMed]
22. Kapadia, S.R.; Makkar, R.; Leon, M.; Abdel-Wahab, M.; Waggoner, T.; Massberg, S.; Rottbauer, W.; Horr, S.; Sondergaard, L.; Karha, J.; et al. Cerebral Embolic Protection during Transcatheter Aortic-Valve Replacement. *N. Engl. J. Med.* **2022**, *387*, 1253–1263. [CrossRef] [PubMed]
23. Majunke, N.; Eplinius, F.; Gutberlet, M.; Moebius-Winkler, S.; Daehnert, I.; Grothoff, M.; Schürer, S.; Mangner, N.; Lurz, P.; Erbs, S. Frequency and clinical course of cerebral embolism in patients undergoing transcatheter left atrial appendage closure. *Eurointervention* **2017**, *13*, 124–130. [CrossRef] [PubMed]

Disclaimer/Publisher's Note: The statements, opinions and data contained in all publications are solely those of the individual author(s) and contributor(s) and not of MDPI and/or the editor(s). MDPI and/or the editor(s) disclaim responsibility for any injury to people or property resulting from any ideas, methods, instructions or products referred to in the content.

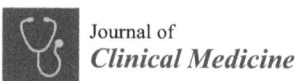
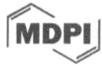

Article

Inducibility of Multiple Ventricular Tachycardia's during a Successful Ablation Procedure Is a Marker of Ventricular Tachycardia Recurrence

Johnatan Nissan [1,2], Avi Sabbag [2,3], Roy Beinart [2,3] and Eyal Nof [2,3,*]

[1] Department of Diagnostic Imaging, Sheba Medical Center, Ramat Gan 52621, Israel; johnatan.n@gmail.com
[2] Sackler School of Medicine, Tel Aviv University, Tel Aviv 69978, Israel; avisabbag@gmail.com (A.S.); roy.beinart@sheba.health.gov.il (R.B.)
[3] Davidai Arrhythmia Center, Leviev Heart Center, Sheba Medical Center, Ramat Gan 52621, Israel
* Correspondence: eyalnof.dr@gmail.com

Abstract: Even after a successful ventricular tachycardia ablation (VTA), some patients have recurrent ventricular tachycardia (VT) during their follow-up. We assessed the long-term predictors of recurrent VT after having a successful VTA. The patients who underwent a successful VTA (defined as the non-inducibility of any VT at the procedure's end) in 2014–2021 at our center in Israel were retrospectively analyzed. A total of 111 successful VTAs were evaluated. Out of them, 31 (27.9%) had a recurrent event of VT after the procedure during a median follow-up time of 264 days. The mean left ventricular ejection fraction (LVEF) was significantly lower among patients with recurrent VT events (28.9 ± 12.67 vs. 23.53 ± 12.224, p = 0.048). A high number of induced VTs (>two) during the procedure was found to be a significant predictor of VT recurrence (24.69% vs. 56.67%, 20 vs. 17, p = 0.002). In a multivariate analysis, a lower LVEF (HR, 0.964; p = 0.037) and a high number of induced VTs (HR, 2.15; p = 0.039) were independent predictors of arrhythmia recurrence. The inducibility of more than two VTs during a VTA procedure remains a predictor of VT recurrence even after a successful VT ablation. This group of patients remains at high risk for VT and should be followed up with and treated more vigorously.

Keywords: ventricular tachycardia; ablation; arrhythmia recurrence

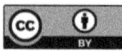

1. Introduction

Ventricular tachycardia ablation (VTA) is a preventive treatment of recurrent ventricular tachycardia (VT) and may reduce mortality among subjects with structural heart disease [1,2]. While the primary endpoint of VTA may be a subject of debate, it is agreed that a minimal endpoint of the non-inducibility of clinical VT is desirable. However, many aim to reach the endpoint of the non-inducibility of any VT. In spite of the above, many patients still experience VT after an ablation. There are several known long-term outcomes predictors, such as VT inducibility at the end of the procedure, being of an older age, having a severely reduced left ventricular ejection fraction (LVEF), and the failure of late potential abolition [1,3–5].

However, there are scarce data on the long-term recurrence of VT after what is deemed a successful VTA. This study aimed to assess the possible predictors of VT recurrence even after achieving the desired endpoint of non-inducibility at the end of the ablation procedure.

2. Material and Methods

2.1. Study Design

This study was approved by the Institutional Review Board of Sheba Medical Center, Tel Hashomer. After retrospectively reviewing a total of 193 procedures, we identified 108 patients who underwent 111 (57.5%) catheter successful ablations of VT between 2014 and 2021 at Davidai Arrhythmia Center at Sheba Medical Center in Israel. Of the other 82 procedures, 19 failed, 27 had partial success, and the inducibility was not checked in the remaining procedures. The data were collected and analyzed in 2021–2022.

2.1.1. Ablation Procedure

Electro-anatomical mapping (EAM) was performed (Carto 3, Biosense Webster, Diamond Bar, CA, USA) using an open irrigated catheter with a 3.5 mm tip (THERMOCOOL SMARTTOUCH™ SF Catheter, Biosense Webster, Diamond Bar, CA, USA). Voltage maps were created during sinus rhythm. Peak-to-peak bipolar electrogram amplitude <0.5 mV was defined as a dense scar, and a voltage of ≥0.5 and <1.5 mV was defined as a scar border zone. Epicardial mapping and ablation were carried out when necessary. EAM was performed with the Pentaray™ Catheter (Biosense Webster, Diamond Bar, CA, USA). Most of the endocardial mapping was performed with a retrograde approach, except 5 cases for which a trans-septal approach was used. In cases in which a epicardial approach was used, the epicardial map was also performed with the Pentaray catheter.

All inducible sustained monomorphic ventricular tachycardias (SMVTs) were targeted for ablation. If VT was mappable, sites were targeted for ablation if pacing entrained the SMVT with concealed fusion and a post-pacing interval (PPI) within 30 ms of the VT cycle length (CL) or by activation mapping. In any case, scar substrate modification was performed. Sites with low-amplitude fractionated electrograms that had long stimulation to QRS, late potentials, or the best-pace map sites were targeted. Pace mapping and entrainment mapping utilized unipolar stimuli with a strength of 10 mA and pulse width of 2 ms Radiofrequency (RF) energy was delivered at a power of 35 to 50 Watts, targeting an impedance drop of at least 10 ohms. The endpoint of all procedures was the non-inducibility of any VT with programmed stimulation (PS) at a basic drive train of 600 and 400 ms with up to 3 extrastimuli. The procedures were performed at a targeted ACT of >300 s. A procedure was defined as successful if the patient was non-inducible for any VT following PS. Partial success was declared when only the clinical VT was no longer inducible, and acute procedural failure was declared if the clinical VT was still inducible.

2.1.2. Study Population

The study's inclusion criteria were patients who underwent VTAs in our institution due to VT events and had a successful VTA procedure. Only patients with inducibility of at least one VT during the procedure were included. All patients were followed up with at our institution, and device interrogation was performed regularly during the follow-up visits (the day after as well as one month, three months, and every six months after the index procedure). Recurrent VT during follow-up was defined as any event of sustained VT (even if self-terminated and tolerable) documented by the patient's implantable cardioverter-defibrillator (ICD) device or in the patient's medical chart. Patients were divided into two groups. Those who had recurrent VT events during follow-up and those who did not. In patients who underwent an additional VTA after the index VTA, the follow-up period evaluated in the study was only the time between the two VTAs.

Each group's main baseline and ablation characteristics were extracted manually from the patient's medical documents. A baseline characteristic was noted if it was defined by the treating physician and was documented in at least two medical documents. Permanent atrial fibrillation (AF) was defined by the 2020 European Society of Cardiology Guidelines for diagnosing and managing atrial fibrillation [6]. Laboratory information was only noted if collected at least 24 h before the procedure, and the closest results to the procedure were assessed. The patients were divided into tertiles by the number of induced VTs during the procedure. The subjects at the highest tertile were categorized as having a "high" number of induced VTs, and the lower two tertiles were categorized as having a "low" number of induced VTs (calculated as a cut-off value of ≥3).

Major complication was defined as one of the following complications: having a cardiac arrest during the operation, post-operative stroke, and pericardial tamponade. A minor complication was defined as a significant groin hematoma (which required treatment with at least one blood unit) or the need for femoral artery intervention.

2.2. Statistical Analysis

The univariate analyses included in this study were the Chi-square test or Fisher's test for categorical variables and the student's t-test for continuous variables. Variables with a calculated p-value ≤ 0.05 in the univariate analyses were included in the multivariate analysis. The multivariate analysis used in the study was Cox regression. The univariate survival analyses used in this study were the Kaplan–Meier curve and the log-rank test. SPSS (version 24.0, IBM, Armonk, NY, USA), R software package (version 4.2.2), and RStudio (version 2023.03.1+446, R Studio PBC, Boston, MA, USA) were used for the statistical analyses in this study.

3. Results

The study included 111 procedures in a total of 108 patients, 30 (27%) of whom had a recurrent VT event after a total median follow-up time of 264 days (IQR, 56–719 days) after the index procedure. A total of 50/111 (45%) had a follow-up time of more than 1 year (either they died or were lost in the follow-up). The median VT-free survival time of the recurrent VT group was 100 days (IQR, 32–529 days), and the median VT-free survival time of the entire cohort was 183 days (IQR, 36–583 days). The 1-year VT recurrence rate of the cohort was 18/50 (36%) among the patients who survived the first year after the procedure and had available data. Out of the 30 patients in the VT recurrence group, 12 (40%) were treated with shock, 14 (46.67%) only with ATP, and 4 (13.33%) were not treated with either shock or ATP.

During the procedure, the mean subject's age was 66.08 ± 9.71 years, and most of the subjects were males (92.8%). Seventy-one (64%) patients had hypertension at baseline, 28 (25.2%) had diabetes mellitus, and 22 (19.8%) had chronic kidney disease. Thirty-seven subjects (33.3%) had a background of AF, 10 had permanent AF, and 27 had non-permanent AF (24.3% and 9%, respectively). Ninety-five (85.6%) subjects had heart failure, without a significant difference between the study's groups (84% vs. 90% for those with non-recurrent VT vs. recurrent VT, respectively). The LVEF was significantly lower in the group of patients who had a VT event after the procedure, compared with that of the group that did not have a VT event (23.53 ± 12.224 vs. 28.9 ± 12.67, respectively, $p = 0.048$). Twenty-eight patients (25.2%) had a history of a previous VTA, without a significant difference between the two groups (25.9% vs. 23.3%; $p = 0.781$). Most patients had ischemic VT etiology (88, 79.3%) and were treated chronically with beta-blockers before the procedure (96, 86.5%) (Table 1).

Table 1. Baseline characteristics: non-VT recurrence group vs. VT recurrence group.

	All ($n = 111$)	Non-VT Recurrence Group ($n = 81$)	VT Recurrence Group ($n = 30$)	p-Value
Age (years)	66.08 ± 9.71	66.57 ± 9.61	64.77 ± 10	NS
Gender (male)	103 (92.8%)	76 (93.8%)	27 (90%)	NS
Hypertension	71 (64%)	53 (65.4%)	18 (60%)	NS
Diabetes mellitus	28 (25.2%)	20 (24.7%)	8 (26.7%)	NS
Heart failure	95 (85.6%)	68 (84%)	27 (90%)	NS
- LVEF	27.45 ± 12.73	28.9 ± 12.67	23.53 ± 12.22	0.048
- LVEF < 30	60 (54.1%)	40 (49.4%)	20 (66.7%)	0.102

Table 1. Cont.

	All (n = 111)	Non-VT Recurrence Group (n = 81)	VT Recurrence Group (n = 30)	p-Value
- LVEF of patients with non-ischemic etiology	35 ± 15.67	37.24 ± 13.55	28.83 ± 20.74	NS
Chronic kidney disease	22 (19.8%)	16 (19.8%)	6 (20%)	NS
Atrial fibrillation	37 (33.3%)	27 (33.3%)	10 (33.3%)	NS
- Non-Permanent	27 (24.3%)	18 (22.2%)	9 (30%)	NS
- Permanent	10 (9%)	9 (11.1%)	1 (3.3%)	0.282
Past VTA	28 (25.2%)	21 (25.9%)	7 (23.3%)	NS
Prior ICD	96 (86.5%)	67 (82.7%)	29 (96.7%)	0.065
Ischemic VT etiology	88 (79.3%)	64 (79%)	24 (80%)	NS
Chronic use of beta-blockers	96 (86.5%)	73 (90.1%)	23 (76.7%)	0.2
Hemoglobin (g/dL)	12.38 ± 1.89	12.45 ± 1.99	12.21 ± 1.65	NS
Platelets count ($\times 10^9$/L)	197.72 ± 66.76	196.89 ± 69.34	199.63 ± 61.65	NS
CRP (mg/L)	39.02 ± 61.86	41.36 ± 64.47	32.35 ± 55.4	NS
Creatinine (mg/dL)	1.23 ± 0.92	1.2 ± 1.04	1.28 ± 0.6	NS

Mean ± standard deviation; VT = ventricular tachycardia; LVEF = left ventricular ejection fraction; VTA = ventricular tachycardia ablation; ICD = implantable cardioverter-defibrillator; CRP = C-reactive protein; NS = not significant, p-value > 0.3.

Thirty-seven (33.33%) procedures were performed with the assistance of an ECMO device, 71 (63.96%) patients were ablated under general anesthesia, and 54 (48.65%) required catecholamines during and after the procedure. The mean number of induced VTs per procedure was 2.27 ± 1.49. The group without VT recurrence had a lower mean of induced VTs than that of the group with VT recurrence (2.12 ± 1.49 vs. 2.67 ± 1.42, respectively, $p = 0.088$; Figure 1).

A high number of induced VTs (>2) was significantly less common in the group which did not have VT recurrence (24.69% vs. 56.67%, 20 vs. 17, respectively, $p = 0.002$). The log-rank test for a high number of induced VTs also indicated this significant association ($p = 0.025$; Figure 2). Forty-seven (42.34%) patients had a posterior-lateral scar, 35 (31.53%) had an antero-septal scar, 17 (15.32%) had a posterior-right scar, 2 (1.8%) had an epicardial scar, and 10 (9.01%) patients did not have a scar (Table 2). The location of the scar did not predict recurrence.

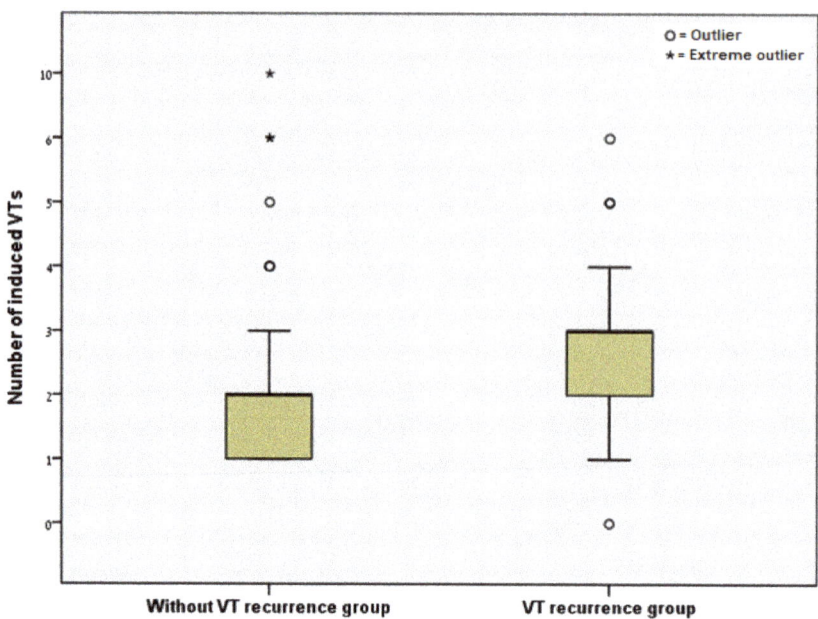

Figure 1. Box plot of the number of induced VTs in the group who did not have VT recurrence vs. the group with VT recurrence ($p = 0.088$). Outlier—3rd quartile + 1.5 × interquartile range or 1st quartile–1.5 × interquartile range; Extreme outlier—3rd quartile + 3 × interquartile range or 1st quartile–3 × interquartile range.

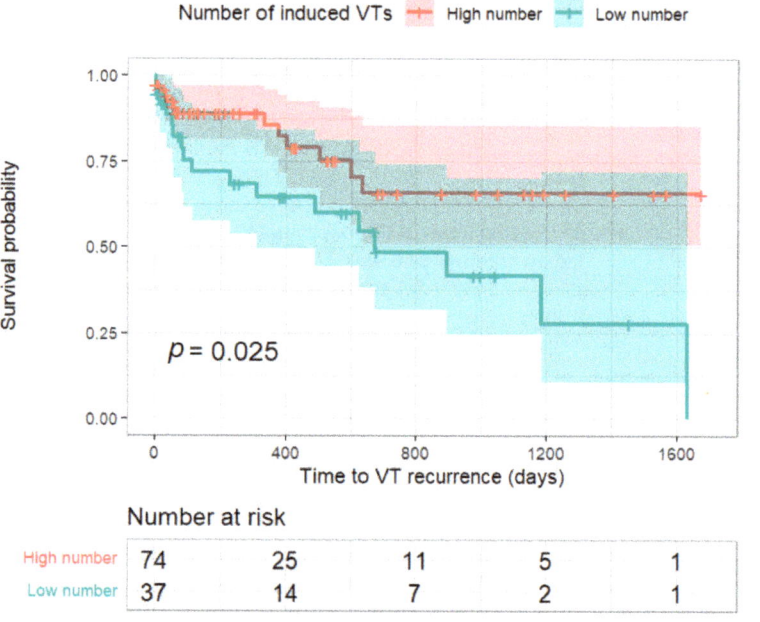

Figure 2. Kaplan–Meier survival curve for a high number of induced VTs during the ablation (p-value = 0.025).

Table 2. Ablation characteristics: non-VT recurrence group vs. VT recurrence group.

	All (n = 111)	Non-VT Recurrence Group (n = 81)	VT Recurrence Group (n = 30)	p-Value
Ablation with ECMO	37 (33.33%)	30 (37.04%)	7 (23.33%)	0.174
General anesthesia	71 (63.96%)	51 (62.96%)	20 (66.66%)	NS
Amines use within 24 h	54 (48.65%)	38 (46.91%)	16 (53.33%)	NS
High number of induced VTs (>2)	37 (33.33%)	20 (24.69%)	17 (56.67%)	0.002
Number of induced VTs	2.27 ± 1.49	2.12 ± 1.49	2.67 ± 1.42	0.088
Scar location				
- Antero-septal	35 (31.53%)	26 (32.1%)	9 (30%)	NS
- Posterior-lateral	47 (42.34%)	33 (40.74%)	14 (46.67%)	NS
- Posterior-right	17 (15.32%)	13 (16.05%)	4 (13.33%)	NS
- Epicardial	2 (1.8%)	0 (0%)	2 (6.67%)	NS
- Without scar	10 (9.01%)	9 (11.11%)	1 (3.33%)	NS

Mean ± standard deviation; VT = ventricular tachycardia; ECMO = extracorporeal membrane oxygenation; NS = not significant, p-value > 0.3.

A total of 85 (76.6%) patients were on anti-arrhythmic medication prior to the procedure. Anti-arrhythmic medications included Amiodarone (64 (57.7%)), Sotalol (19 (17.1%)), and Mexiletine (19 (17.1%)). Out of this patient group, 94 (84.7%) were discharged on the same anti-arrhythmic medication, and 17 (15.3%) were discharged on another anti-arrhythmic medication. This did not differ between groups (10 (12.3%) vs. 7 (23.3%); $p = 0.233$).

Post-ablation major complications were observed in two (1.8%) patients and minor complications in two (1.8%) patients. The prevalence of any type of complication did not differ between groups. Seventeen (15.32%) patients died during the follow-up time: nine (11.11%) patients in the group that did not have VT recurrence and eight (26.67%) patients in the VT recurrence group ($p = 0.071$). The mean mortality time after ablation was 421.94 ± 554.92 days (172.44 ± 361.93 days in the group that did not have VT recurrence, and 702.62 ± 619.75 days in the VT recurrence group ($p = 0.045$)) (Table 3).

Table 3. Ablation outcomes: non-VT recurrence group vs. VT recurrence group.

	All (n = 111)	Non-VT Recurrence Group (n = 81)	VT Recurrence Group (n = 30)	p-Value
Major complications	2 (1.8%)	2 (2.47%)	0 (0%)	NS
Minor complications	2 (1.8%)	1 (1.23%)	1 (3.33%)	NS
Mortality	17 (15.32%)	9 (11.11%)	8 (26.67%)	0.071
- Time to mortality (days)	421.94 ± 554.92	172.44 ± 361.93	702.62 ± 619.75	0.045

Mean ± standard deviation; VT = ventricular tachycardia; NS = not significant, p-value > 0.3.

In the multivariate Cox regression analysis, the LVEF (Hazard ratio [HR], 0.964; 95% confidence interval [95% CI], 0.932–0.998; $p = 0.037$) and a high number of induced VTs (HR, 2.15; 95% CI, 1.04–4.45; $p = 0.039$) were significant predictors of VT recurrence (Table 4).

Table 4. Multivariate Cox regression of the risk for VT recurrence.

	HR (95% CI)	p-Value
LVEF *	0.964 (0.93–1)	0.037
High vs. low number of induced VTs	2.15 (1.04–4.45)	0.039

* LVEF as a continuous variable; VT = ventricular tachycardia; HR = hazard ratio; CI = confidence interval; LVEF = left ventricular ejection fraction.

4. Discussion

To the best of our knowledge, this is the first study to separately analyze the predictors of VT recurrence after what is acutely considered a successful VTA. Although several predictors for VT recurrence have been described previously in the literature, these studies did not characterize this specific sub-group of patients, which is typically considered a lower-risk group for VT recurrence and mortality [3,7]. Our study indicates two possible predictors for VT recurrence after a successful VTA—a lower LVEF and a high number of induced VTs during the procedure.

Although a lower LVEF [8–13] and a high number of induced VTs during ablation [9,12,14] have been previously described as predictors of VT recurrence after VTA, our data are unique in the fact that these variables remain as predictors even after a successful VTA. This finding is surprising as, at the end of the procedure, all our patients by definition were non-inducible for any VT. Thus, the substrate creating the inducible VT seen at the beginning of the procedure was considered as successfully targeted. In spite of the above, these patients had a higher VT recurrence rate, most probably reflecting the presence of a more complex substrate.

The predictors demonstrated in our study can serve as a possible indicator for the unknown underlying mechanism through which VTs are developed after a successful VTA. As a lower LVEF has already been assessed as a predictor of VTA in the study of Haanschoten et al. [8], it was hypothesized that the underlying mechanism might be related to a possible more extensive and complex arrhythmogenic substrate in patients with a lower LVEF, which can disrupt the elimination of all the possible arrhythmogenic pathways during the procedure. Furthermore, de Riva et al. [9] suggested that not all VTs have a fixed reentry mechanism, especially among patients with enhanced cardiac remodeling and heart failure, which might generate additional focal reentry cycles that are not accurately reproducible by programmed electric stimulation. In our study, only those with non-inducible VTAs at the conclusion of the procedure were included, indicating that all the "fixed" arrhythmogenic pathways were probably not inducible at the end of the ablation. This might strengthen the hypothesis of focal arrhythmic mechanisms that generate VT recurrence, foci that electric stimulation could not generate during the procedure. The same hypothesis can also be implicated by the second predictor found in the study—a high number of induced VTs. A higher number of induced VTs may indicate a more complex scar substrate tissue which may prevent the stimulation of these focal or even reentrant pathways.

An alternative explanation could be a deeper (intramural) substrate that was not mapped or recognized during the procedure. Previous studies [15,16] have found that intramural substrates account for a relatively large number of VTs, even in ischemic cardiomyopathy patients. This intramural substrate could be identified mainly during VT by electro-anatomical mapping. If the VT arising from such a substrate is non-inducible during the procedure, it might be challenging to identify the substrate and target it.

The main clinical implication of our study is that patients with more than two inducible VTs during a VTA procedure should be followed up rigorously and anti-arrhythmic medication should most probably be continued even if it is a successful procedure. Further studies should assess the possible underlying mechanism of VT recurrence among patients who underwent a successful VTA to evaluate the causes of VT recurrence after a VTA.

The current analysis indicates a 36% one-year VT recurrence rate after a successful VTA. Comparisons to previous studies' outcomes are relatively limited due to the lack of standardization in the outcome time. Breitenstein et al. [17] recently assessed the one-year recurrence rate of VT after a successful VTA as 45% in a large cohort of patients with structural heart diseases, and Okubo et al. [18] evaluated it was 16% among patients with a late potential abolition and 32% without one. Other studies with relatively small non-inducibility study groups evaluated this recurrence rate as 0–40% among patients with various clinical characteristics [9,11,19,20]. The high recurrence rate heterogeneity might be related to the lack of study population uniformity and different patient baseline characteristics.

Our study's main limitation is the demonstration of a causal link only between successful VTA characteristics and VT recurrence without investigating the underlying reason for this association. Further studies should assess the mechanism of this association. Another limitation is the study's retrospective design which might include natural retrospective biases, such as information and selection biases, and the relatively low number of patients, which might fail to recognize other predictors.

5. Conclusions

The inducibility of many VTs during a VTA procedure predicts VT events in the long term, even if the patient is deemed non-inducible for any VT at the termination of the procedure.

Author Contributions: Conceptualization: E.N.; methodology: J.N. and A.S.; formal analysis and investigation: J.N., E.N. and A.S.; writing—original draft preparation: J.N. and E.N.; writing—review and editing: E.N. and R.B.; supervision: E.N. and R.B. All authors have read and agreed to the published version of the manuscript.

Funding: This research received no external funding.

Institutional Review Board Statement: The study was conducted according to the guidelines of the Declaration of Helsinki and approved by the Institutional Review Board of Sheba Medical Center, Tel Hashomer, institutional approved code: SMC-4803-17.

Informed Consent Statement: The study included a retrospective analysis of existing hospital data and was approved by the Institutional Review Board.

Data Availability Statement: Anonymized data are available on request from the corresponding author.

Conflicts of Interest: The authors declare no conflict of interest.

References

1. Della Bella, P.; Baratto, F.; Tsiachris, D.; Trevisi, N.; Vergara, P.; Bisceglia, C.; Petracca, F.; Carbucicchio, C.; Benussi, S.; Maisano, F.; et al. Management of Ventricular Tachycardia in the Setting of a Dedicated Unit for the Treatment of Complex Ventricular Arrhythmias: Long-Term Outcome after Ablation. *Circulation* **2013**, *127*, 1359–1368. [CrossRef] [PubMed]
2. Tung, R.; Vaseghi, M.; Frankel, D.S.; Vergara, P.; Di Biase, L.; Nagashima, K.; Yu, R.; Vangala, S.; Tseng, C.-H.; Choi, E.-K.; et al. Freedom from Recurrent Ventricular Tachycardia after Catheter Ablation Is Associated with Improved Survival in Patients with Structural Heart Disease: An International VT Ablation Center Collaborative Group Study. *Heart Rhythm* **2015**, *12*, 1997–2007. [CrossRef] [PubMed]
3. Silberbauer, J.; Oloriz, T.; Maccabelli, G.; Tsiachris, D.; Baratto, F.; Vergara, P.; Mizuno, H.; Bisceglia, C.; Marzi, A.; Sora, N.; et al. Noninducibility and Late Potential Abolition: A Novel Combined Prognostic Procedural End Point for Catheter Ablation of Postinfarction Ventricular Tachycardia. *Circ. Arrhythm. Electrophysiol.* **2014**, *7*, 424–435. [CrossRef] [PubMed]
4. Tilz, R.R.; Lin, T.; Eckardt, L.; Deneke, T.; Andresen, D.; Wieneke, H.; Brachmann, J.; Kääb, S.; Chun, K.R.J.; Münkler, P.; et al. Ablation Outcomes and Predictors of Mortality Following Catheter Ablation for Ventricular Tachycardia: Data from the German Multicenter Ablation Registry. *J. Am. Heart Assoc.* **2018**, *7*, e007045. [CrossRef] [PubMed]
5. Della Bella, P.; Riva, S.; Fassini, G.; Giraldi, F.; Berti, M.; Klersy, C.; Trevisi, N. Incidence and Significance of Pleomorphism in Patients with Postmyocardial Infarction Ventricular Tachycardia. Acute and Long-Term Outcome of Radiofrequency Catheter Ablation. *Eur. Heart J.* **2004**, *25*, 1127–1138. [CrossRef] [PubMed]
6. Hindricks, G.; Potpara, T.; Dagres, N.; Arbelo, E.; Bax, J.J.; Blomström-Lundqvist, C.; Boriani, G.; Castella, M.; Dan, G.-A.; Dilaveris, P.E.; et al. 2020 ESC Guidelines for the Diagnosis and Management of Atrial Fibrillation Developed in Collaboration with the European Association for Cardio-Thoracic Surgery (EACTS). *Eur. Heart J.* **2021**, *42*, 373–498. [CrossRef] [PubMed]

7. Ghanbari, H.; Baser, K.; Yokokawa, M.; Stevenson, W.; Della Bella, P.; Vergara, P.; Deneke, T.; Kuck, K.-H.; Kottkamp, H.; Fei, S.; et al. Noninducibility in Postinfarction Ventricular Tachycardia as an End Point for Ventricular Tachycardia Ablation and Its Effects on Outcomes: A Meta-Analysis. *Circ. Arrhythm. Electrophysiol.* **2014**, *7*, 677–683. [CrossRef] [PubMed]
8. Haanschoten, D.M.; Smit, J.J.J.; Adiyaman, A.; Ramdat Misier, A.R.; HM Delnoy, P.P.; Elvan, A. Long-Term Outcome of Catheter Ablation in Post-Infarction Recurrent Ventricular Tachycardia. *Scand. Cardiovasc. J.* **2019**, *53*, 62–70. [CrossRef] [PubMed]
9. de Riva, M.; Piers, S.R.D.; Kapel, G.F.L.; Watanabe, M.; Venlet, J.; Trines, S.A.; Schalij, M.J.; Zeppenfeld, K. Reassessing Noninducibility as Ablation Endpoint of Post-Infarction Ventricular Tachycardia. *Circ. Arrhythm. Electrophysiol.* **2015**, *8*, 853–862. [CrossRef] [PubMed]
10. Vergara, P.; Tzou, W.S.; Tung, R.; Brombin, C.; Nonis, A.; Vaseghi, M.; Frankel, D.S.; Di Biase, L.; Tedrow, U.; Mathuria, N.; et al. Predictive Score for Identifying Survival and Recurrence Risk Profiles in Patients Undergoing Ventricular Tachycardia Ablation. *Circ. Arrhythm. Electrophysiol.* **2018**, *11*, e006730. [CrossRef] [PubMed]
11. Piers, S.R.D.; Leong, D.P.; van Taxis, C.F.B.; Tayyebi, M.; Trines, S.A.; Pijnappels, D.A.; Delgado, V.; Schalij, M.J.; Zeppenfeld, K. Outcome of Ventricular Tachycardia Ablation in Patients with Nonischemic Cardiomyopathy. *Circ. Arrhythm. Electrophysiol.* **2013**, *6*, 513–521. [CrossRef] [PubMed]
12. Naruse, Y.; de Riva, M.; Watanabe, M.; Wijnmaalen, A.P.; Venlet, J.; Timmer, M.; Schalij, M.J.; Zeppenfeld, K. The Prognostic Value of J-wave Pattern for Recurrence of Ventricular Tachycardia after Catheter Ablation in Patients with Myocardial Infarction. *Pacing Clin. Electrophysiol.* **2021**, *44*, 657–666. [CrossRef] [PubMed]
13. Quinto, L.; Sanchez-Somonte, P.; Alarcón, F.; Garre, P.; Castillo, À.; San Antonio, R.; Borras, R.; Guasch, E.; Arbelo, E.; Tolosana, J.M.; et al. Ventricular Tachycardia Burden Reduction after Substrate Ablation: Predictors of Recurrence. *Heart Rhythm* **2021**, *18*, 896–904. [CrossRef] [PubMed]
14. Tung, R.; Josephson, M.E.; Reddy, V.; Reynolds, M.R.; SMASH-VT Investigators. Influence of Clinical and Procedural Predictors on Ventricular Tachycardia Ablation Outcomes: An Analysis from the Substrate Mapping and Ablation in Sinus Rhythm to Halt Ventricular Tachycardia Trial (SMASH-VT). *J. Cardiovasc. Electrophysiol.* **2010**, *21*, 799–803. [CrossRef] [PubMed]
15. Bhaskaran, A.; Nayyar, S.; Porta-Sánchez, A.; Jons, C.; Massé, S.; Magtibay, K.; Aukhojee, P.; Ha, A.; Bokhari, M.; Tung, R.; et al. Direct and Indirect Mapping of Intramural Space in Ventricular Tachycardia. *Heart Rhythm* **2020**, *17*, 439–446. [CrossRef] [PubMed]
16. Kotake, Y.; Nalliah, C.J.; Campbell, T.; Bennett, R.G.; Turnbull, S.; Kumar, S. Comparison of the Arrhythmogenic Substrate for Ventricular Tachycardia in Patients with Ischemic vs Non-Ischemic Cardiomyopathy—Insights from High-Density, Multi-Electrode Catheter Mapping. *J. Interv. Card. Electrophysiol.* **2023**, *66*, 5–14. [CrossRef] [PubMed]
17. Breitenstein, A.; Sawhney, V.; Providencia, R.; Honarbakhsh, S.; Ullah, W.; Dhinoja, M.B.; Schilling, R.J.; Babu, G.G.; Chow, A.; Lambiase, P.; et al. Ventricular Tachycardia Ablation in Structural Heart Disease: Impact of Ablation Strategy and Non-Inducibility as an End-Point on Long Term Outcome. *Int. J. Cardiol.* **2019**, *277*, 110–117. [CrossRef] [PubMed]
18. Okubo, K.; Gigli, L.; Trevisi, N.; Foppoli, L.; Radinovic, A.; Bisceglia, C.; Frontera, A.; D'Angelo, G.; Cireddu, M.; Paglino, G.; et al. Long-Term Outcome After Ventricular Tachycardia Ablation in Nonischemic Cardiomyopathy: Late Potential Abolition and VT Noninducibility. *Circ. Arrhythm. Electrophysiol.* **2020**, *13*, e008307. [CrossRef] [PubMed]
19. Kapel, G.F.L.; Reichlin, T.; Wijnmaalen, A.P.; Piers, S.R.D.; Holman, E.R.; Tedrow, U.B.; Schalij, M.J.; Stevenson, W.G.; Zeppenfeld, K. Re-Entry Using Anatomically Determined Isthmuses. *Circ. Arrhythm. Electrophysiol.* **2015**, *8*, 102–109. [CrossRef] [PubMed]
20. Berte, B.; Sacher, F.; Venlet, J.; Andreu, D.; Mahida, S.; Aldhoon, B.; De Potter, T.; Sarkozy, A.; Tavernier, R.; Andronache, M.; et al. VT Recurrence After Ablation: Incomplete Ablation or Disease Progression? A Multicentric European Study. *J. Cardiovasc. Electrophysiol.* **2016**, *27*, 80–87. [CrossRef] [PubMed]

Disclaimer/Publisher's Note: The statements, opinions and data contained in all publications are solely those of the individual author(s) and contributor(s) and not of MDPI and/or the editor(s). MDPI and/or the editor(s) disclaim responsibility for any injury to people or property resulting from any ideas, methods, instructions or products referred to in the content.

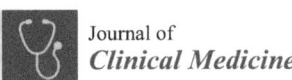

Article

Complicated Pocket Infection in Patients Undergoing Lead Extraction: Characteristics and Outcomes

Anat Milman [1,2,*,†], Anat Wieder-Finesod [2,3,†], Guy Zahavi [2,4], Amit Meitus [2], Saar Kariv [2], Yuval Shafir [1,2], Roy Beinart [1,2], Galia Rahav [2,3] and Eyal Nof [1,2]

1. Leviev Heart Institute, The Chaim Sheba Medical Center, Tel Hashomer, Ramat Gan 5262000, Israel; eyalnof.dr@gmail.com (E.N.)
2. Sackler School of Medicine, Tel Aviv University, Tel Aviv 6997801, Israel; anat.wieder@sheba.health.gov.il (A.W.-F.)
3. The Infectious Diseases Unit, Sheba Medical Center, Tel-Hashomer, Ramat Gan 5262000, Israel
4. Department of Anesthesiology and Intensive Care, The Chaim Sheba Medical Center, Tel Hashomer, Ramat Gan 5262000, Israel
* Correspondence: anatmilman@gmail.com
† These authors contributed equally to this work.

Abstract: Cardiac implantable electronic device (CIED) infection can present with pocket or systemic manifestations, both necessitating complete device removal and pathogen-directed antimicrobial therapy. Here, we aim to characterize those presenting with both pocket and systemic infection. A retrospective analysis of CIED extraction procedures included 300 patients divided into isolated pocket (n = 104, 34.7%), complicated pocket (n = 54, 18%), and systemic infection (n = 142, 47.3%) groups. The systemic and complicated pocket groups frequently presented with leukocytosis and fever > 37.8, as opposed to the isolated pocket group. *Staphylococcus aureus* was the most common pathogen in the systemic and complicated pocket groups (43.7% and 31.5%, respectively), while Coagulase-negative staphylococci (CONS) predominated (31.7%) in the isolated pocket group (10.6%, $p < 0.001$). No differences were observed in procedural success or complications rates. Kaplan–Meier survival analysis found that at three years of follow-up, the rate of all-cause mortality was significantly higher among patients with systemic infection compared to both pocket groups ($p < 0.001$), with the curves diverging at thirty days. In this study, we characterize a new entity of complicated pocket infection. Despite the systemic pattern of infection, their prognosis is similar to isolated pocket infection. We suggest that this special category be presented separately in future publications of CIED infections.

Keywords: cardiac implantable electronic device; transvenous lead extraction; infection

1. Introduction

Over the past decade, there has been a dramatic increase in the number of cardiac implantable electronic devices (CIED) [1,2]. As a result, an exponential rise in transvenous lead extraction (TLE) procedures has evolved. TLE has exceeded the increase in implantation rates [3–7].

Infection is a serious complication after CIED implantation [1], necessitating complete device removal and pathogen-directed antimicrobial drug therapy [2]. Infections from CIEDs are costly, associated with substantial in-hospital and long-term mortality [3]. Optimal management of CIED infection at initial presentation is critical to reduce infection-associated morbidity, mortality, hospital length of stay, and relapse [4,7].

CIED infections can have different presentations. Classically, patients are divided into pocket vs. systemic infection [8]. Pocket infection typically presents with inflammatory changes at the pocket site, including erythema, swelling, pain, warmth, drainage, purulence, erosion, and dehiscence. Pocket infection may involve intravascular or intracardiac portions

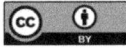

of leads, and if this situation results in bacteremia, lead infection, or endocarditis, systemic symptoms are prominent as well. The majority of patients present within 12 months of device placement or revision [9]. The pathogenesis is seeding of the pathogen from the skin to the generator. Systemic infection, on the other hand, presents with a primary bloodstream infection (bacteremia, lead infection, or endocarditis), without signs of pocket infection. The suggested mechanism is hematogenous seeding of device leads or heart valves from a distant source of bacteremia. Diagnosis of systemic CIED infections can be challenging and is often delayed [10,11].

Staphylococcal species are responsible for 60–80% of CIED infections [10,11]. *Staphylococcus aureus* is a notably virulent bacterium accounting for 25% of CIED infections, which often result in acute onset of fever and rigors. Coagulase-negative staphylococcus is the most common cause of device pocket-related infection but is less virulent and has fewer systemic symptoms [12,13]. Gram-negative bacilli account for 6–10%, while other Gram-positive pathogens, fungi, and skin flora account for an even lesser percentage. The pathogenesis of the CIED infection influences the microbiology and the clinical outcome.

Both pocket infections that are complicated with systemic infection and systemic infections without pocket infection may result in systemic inflammatory response syndrome (SIRS) criteria (fever or hypothermia, tachycardia, tachypnea, and leukocytosis or leukopenia) and/or hypotension (systolic blood pressure < 90 mm Hg or a >40 mm Hg drop from baseline). The aim of this study is to characterize those with complicated pocket infections, since these patients are not well-characterized, and compare them to patients with systemic only and pocket only CIED infections.

2. Methods

A retrospective analysis of all consecutive CIED extraction procedures at the Sheba Medical Center from July 2010 to December 2018 was performed. Demographic, clinical, laboratory, imaging, and microbiologic data were extracted from each chart. Device removal and associated complications were documented.

2.1. TLE Procedure

All TLE procedures were performed with a cardiothoracic surgeon immediately available on site. Patients were under general anesthesia, with hemodynamic monitoring. A large-bore femoral venous access was inserted in all patients. The procedure was performed by qualified experienced operators. A stepwise approach was used in all patients, as previously described by our group [14]. The TLE procedure was terminated after complete removal of the leads, or when lead fragments could not be removed or in the event of a major complication.

Complications were divided into major complications (defined as those that threaten life, such as tamponade, required surgical intervention, or resulted in death). Complications that did not meet the major complication criteria were classified as minor complications.

Success or failure was defined by the radiological findings, not clinical. Patients were divided into three groups depending on the outcome of the extraction procedure:
1. 'Complete success' was classified as the removal of the entire lead system.
2. 'Partial success' was defined as when most of the lead was removed, leaving at most 4 cm of coil and/or insulation and/or lead tip.
3. 'Failure' was defined if more than ≥4 cm of the tip remained.

All extraction patient records were reviewed and procedures due to infection were identified. Inclusion criteria were all patients undergoing extraction due to CIED-related infections, either carrying a permanent pacemaker (PPM) or implantable cardioverter defibrillator (ICD). Out of these, only records with confirmed culture growth, either pocket, blood, and/or lead cultures, were included in the study population. Patient data were collected and analyzed in accordance with the Sheba Helsinki Committee authorization for this study.

Outcome data were collected from records of follow-up visits to our outpatient clinic or hospitalization records. Due to the large volume of patients referred from other medical centers solely for extraction, some patients were not included in the follow-up. Mortality data were extracted from an Israeli governmental registry; thus, mortality rates were accurate for all patients, regardless of clinical follow-up.

For the purpose of this analysis, patients were firstly divided into pocket and systemic CIED infection, and then further divided into three groups:

Isolated pocket infection: Infection limited to the CIED pocket, such as localized cellulitis, swelling, discharge, dehiscence, or pain, with or without signs of fever. These patients have negative blood cultures and no evidence of a lead/valve vegetation on transesophageal echocardiogram (TEE).

Complicated pocket infection: pocket infection with positive blood cultures consistent with CIED infection or lead/valve vegetation seen on echocardiography.

Systemic infection: bacteremia or vegetations without signs or symptoms of pocket infection, including CIED-associated native or prosthetic valve endocarditis (CIED-IE) with no signs of generator pocket infection.

The following pathogen groups were predefined for analysis: *Staphylococcus aureus* (SA), Coagulase-negative staphylococcus (CONS), *Streptococcus* spp., *Enterococcus* spp., *Pseudomonas aeruginosa*, Enterobacteriaceae (*Escherichia coli*, *Citrobacter koseri*, *Klebsiella* spp., and more), and skin flora bacteria (*Corynebacterium* spp., *Cutibacterium* (formerly *Propionibacterium*) *acnes*), Candida, and mixed bacteria.

2.2. Principles of Antimicrobial Therapy

The duration and type of antimicrobial therapy was based on the infection group (isolated pocket, complicated pocket, and systemic) and culture results with susceptibility testing. The main recommendations following CIED removal were, for isolated pocket infections: treatment of 10 to 14 days with IV or PO antimicrobials, with a longer duration for deep wounds and wounds that underwent extra debridement and surgical procedures. Complicated pocket infections were treated according to the infection characteristics: infections with positive blood cultures and/or valve vegetations were treated for 6 weeks. Infections with lead vegetations and negative blood cultures, and no involvement of other cardiac structures by echocardiography, were treated for 4 weeks with IV or PO antimicrobials (or oral switch after starting IV), depending on the specific pathogen. Systemic infections were treated for 6 weeks with IV therapy. Specific treatment regimens were as recommended by the guidelines [1,2,15].

2.3. Statistical Analysis

Continuous variables are shown as mean ± SD or as median (IQR), and categorical variables as n (%). Variables were compared with an ANOVA test, Kruskal–Wallis test, or a Pearson's chi-squared test. The survival probability at specific time points was estimated with logistic regression. All predictors with a significant hazard ratio or odds ratio (p-value ≤ 0.05) in univariate analysis were included in multivariate prediction models. For variables included in multivariate models, missing data were imputed if at least 75% of the data were complete. Missing data about medical diagnoses and procedural complications were marked as 'No'. Kaplan–Meier survival curves were compared using the log-rank test. Significant p-values were considered when $p < 0.05$. All statistical analyses were conducted with R version 3.6.1 from R Foundation for Statistical Computing (Vienna, Austria).

3. Results

3.1. Demographic, Clinical, and Device Data

3.1.1. Patient Characteristics

A total of 300 patients were eligible for the study. Baseline characteristics are shown in Table 1. Out of those, 158 (52.7%) had a pocket infection (divided into 104 (65.8%) isolated pocket infections and 54 (34.2%) complicated) and 142 (47.3%) had a systemic infection which did not involve the pocket. In the entire cohort, most of the patients were males, with a mean age of 66.6 ± 15.5 years at the time of extraction. Their comorbidities and lab results are listed in Table 1. More than half of the extracted devices were pacemakers (59.7%), followed by cardiac resynchronization therapy defibrillators (CRTD) (24.7%), implantable cardiac defibrillators (ICD) (12.7%), and cardiac resynchronization therapy pacemakers (CRTP) (3%).

Table 1. Baseline characteristics of the study group.

Infection Type		Overall	Pocket Infection Isolated	Pocket Infection Complicated	Systemic	p Value
Number of patients		300	104	54	142	
Demographics						
	Female	67 (22.3)	22 (21.2)	11 (20.4)	34 (23.9)	0.812
	Age (mean ± SD)	66.6 ± 15.5	66.6 ± 16.6	64.2 ± 18.8	67.5 ± 13.0	0.414
Referral from other center		205 (68.3)	71 (68.3)	35 (64.8)	99 (69.7)	0.805
Comorbiditis						
	Smoking	78 (26.0)	25 (24.0)	14 (25.9)	39 (27.5)	0.833
	Atrial fibrillation	110 (36.7)	40 (38.5)	13 (24.1)	57 (40.1)	0.102
	Hypertension	180 (60.0)	62 (59.6)	26 (48.1)	92 (64.8)	0.104
	Heart failure	135 (45.0)	44 (42.3)	26 (48.1)	65 (45.8)	0.758
	Stroke	42 (14.0)	14 (13.5)	4 (7.4)	24 (16.9)	0.227
	Vascular disease	168 (56.0)	58 (55.8)	27 (50.0)	83 (58.5)	0.566
	Malignancy	21 (7.0)	8 (7.7)	3 (5.6)	10 (7.0)	0.882
	Diabetes mellitus	131 (43.7)	35 (33.7)	19 (35.2)	77 (54.2)	0.002
	LVEF (%±SD)	40.5 ± 16.5	40.7 ± 15.4	39.4 ± 17.1	40.8 ± 17.2	0.878
Prosthetic valve						0.061
	Biological	14 (4.7)	2 (1.9)	1 (1.9)	11 (7.7)	
	Mechanical	15 (5.0)	6 (5.8)	5 (9.3)	4 (2.8)	
	No	271 (90.3)	96 (92.3)	48 (88.9)	127 (89.4)	
Device type						0.546
	CRT-D	74 (24.7)	29 (27.9)	13 (24.1)	32 (22.5)	
	CRT-P	9 (3.0)	4 (3.8)	3 (5.6)	2 (1.4)	
	ICD	38 (12.7)	14 (13.5)	8 (14.8)	16 (11.3)	
	PM	179 (59.7)	57 (54.8)	30 (55.6)	92 (64.8)	

Abbreviations: LVEF—left ventricular ejection fraction; CRT—resynchronization therapy; PM—pacemaker; ICD—implantable cardiac defibrillator.

The only differences in comorbidities that were observed between the groups included a significantly higher prevalence of diabetes (54.2%) in the systemic infection group compared to both pocket infection groups (33.7% and 35.2%) (Table 1).

Prosthetic valves were found in 9.7% of the patients. In patients with a systemic infection, 7.7% had a biologic prosthetic valve and 2.8% had a mechanical valve. In both pocket infection groups, mechanical valves were more prevalent than biological valves (5.8% isolated and 9.3% complicated, and 1.9% isolated and 1.9% complicated, respectively).

No difference was observed in the type of device extracted between all three groups (Table 1).

3.1.2. Infection Manifestation

All groups had a similar rate of history of prior infection (Table 2). The prevalence of temperature higher than 37.8 °C was significantly different between all 3 groups (71.8% in the systemic infection group vs. 42.6% in the complicated pocket infection group vs. 8.7% in the isolated pocket infection group; $p < 0.001$) (Table 2). Leukocytosis was also more prevalent in the systemic group and the complicated pocket group compared to the isolated pocket infection group (50% vs. 35.2% vs. 22.1%, respectively, $p < 0.001$). Duration of antibiotic treatment was significantly longer for both the systemic and complicated pocket infection groups compared to the isolated pocket group (Table 2).

Table 2. Infection manifestation.

Infection Type		Overall	Pocket Isolated	Pocket Complicated	Systemic	p Value
Number of patients		300	104	54	142	
Prior device infection		44 (14.7)	19 (18.3)	9 (16.7)	16 (11.3)	0.278
Temperature > 37.8 °C						<0.001
	No	156 (52.0)	94 (90.4)	28 (51.9)	34 (23.9)	
	Yes	134 (44.7)	9 (8.7)	23 (42.6)	102 (71.8)	
	Unspecified	10 (3.3)	1 (1.0)	3 (5.6)	6 (4.2)	
Lekuocytosis > 10K		113 (37.7)	23 (22.1)	19 (35.2)	71 (50.0)	<0.001
Duration of antibiotics (days)		27.7 ± 19.8	16.5 ± 11.5	32.1 ± 24.6	34.1 ± 19.3	<0.001
Lab results						
	Creatinine (mg/dL)	1.4 ± 1.0	1.2 ± 0.7	1.3 ± 0.8	1.6 ± 1.1	0.001
	Hemoglobin (g/dL)	11.1 ± 1.9	12.0 ± 1.7	11.9 ± 1.5	10.2 ± 1.6	<0.001
	Albumin (g/dL)	3.2 ± 0.7	3.7 ± 0.5	3.5 ± 0.5	2.8 ± 0.7	<0.001
Pocket Dehiscence						<0.001
	Negative	179 (59.7)	25 (24.0)	15 (27.8)	139 (97.9)	
	Positive	117 (39.0)	78 (75.0)	39 (72.2)	0 (0.0)	
	Unspecified	4 (1.3)	1 (1.0)	0 (0.0)	3 (2.1)	
Pocket Culture						<0.001
	Negative	130 (43.3)	15 (14.4)	5 (9.3)	110 (77.5)	
	Positive	154 (51.3)	87 (83.7)	48 (88.9)	19 (13.4)	
	Not performed	10 (3.3)	0 (0.0)	0 (0.0)	10 (7.0)	
	Unspecified	6 (2.0)	2 (1.9)	1 (1.9)	3 (2.1)	
Blood Culture						<0.001
	Negative	149 (49.7)	102 (98.1)	24 (44.4)	23 (16.2)	
	Positive	148 (49.3)	0 (0.0)	29 (53.7)	119 (83.8)	
	Not performed	2 (0.7)	1 (1.0)	1 (1.9)	0 (0.0)	
	Unspecified	1 (0.3)	1 (1.0)	0 (0.0)	0 (0.0)	
Lead Culture						0.501
	Negative	205 (68.3)	67 (64.4)	39 (72.2)	99 (69.7)	
	Positive	85 (28.3)	31 (29.8)	14 (25.9)	40 (28.2)	
	Not performed	8 (2.7)	5 (4.8)	1 (1.9)	2 (1.4)	
	Unspecified	2 (0.7)	1 (1.0)	0 (0.0)	1 (0.7)	
Transthoracic Echocardiography						0.002
	No vegetation	166 (55.3)	61 (58.7)	34 (63.0)	71 (50.0)	
	Vegetation	25 (8.3)	0 (0.0)	9 (16.7)	16 (11.3)	
	Not performed	69 (23.0)	21 (20.2)	10 (18.5)	38 (26.8)	
	Unspecified	40 (13.3)	22 (21.2)	1 (1.9)	17 (12.0)	
Transesophageal Echocardiography						<0.001
	No vegetation	75 (25.0)	40 (38.5)	12 (22.2)	23 (16.2)	
	Vegetation	102 (34.0)	0 (0.0)	28 (51.9)	74 (52.1)	
	Not performed	29 (9.7)	22 (21.2)	3 (5.6)	4 (2.8)	
	Unspecified	94 (31.3)	42 (40.4)	11 (20.4)	41 (28.9)	

Patients with a systemic infection were sicker, as demonstrated by their lab results: higher creatinine (1.6 ± 1.1 mg/dL, $p = 0.001$), lower hemoglobin (10.2 ± 1.6 g/dL, $p < 0.001$), and lower albumin (2.8 ± 0.7 g/dL, $p < 0.001$). As expected, the complicated pocket infection group's lab results were worse than those in the isolated pocket infection group (Table 2).

Positive pocket cultures were found in majority of both pocket infection groups (83.7% in the isolated and 88.9% in the complicated pocket infection groups) (Table 2). Positive blood cultures were more common in the systemic group (83.8%) than the complicated pocket group (53.7%) ($p < 0.001$). Positive lead cultures were relatively rare in all groups (mean 28.3%, $p = 0.501$).

Lead or valve vegetations were found in 28 patients (51.9%) of the complicated pocket group and in 74 patients (52.1%) of the systemic group. Most vegetations were demonstrated by transesophageal echocardiography (TEE) and not by transthoracic echocardiography (TTE) (TEE—52.1% and 51.9% for systemic and complicated pocket infection groups vs. TTE—11.3% and 16.7%, respectively; $p < 0.001$) (Table 2).

3.1.3. Infectious Pathogens

SA was the most common pathogen responsible for CIED infection in the systemic and complicated pocket infection groups (43.7% and 31.5% vs. 10.6% in the isolated pocket group patients; $p < 0.001$), while CONS was more frequent in the isolated pocket infection group (31.7% vs. 11.1% in the complicated pocket group and 10.6% in the systemic group; $p < 0.001$, Figure 1). Gram-negative pathogens (especially pseudomonas) were more frequent in both pocket groups (15.4% in the isolated and 29.6% in the complicated pocket groups) compared to the systemic group (7.7%). CONS and skin pathogens were more frequent in the isolated pocket group (37.5% vs. 13% in the complicated pocket group and 12% in the systemic group) (Figure 1).

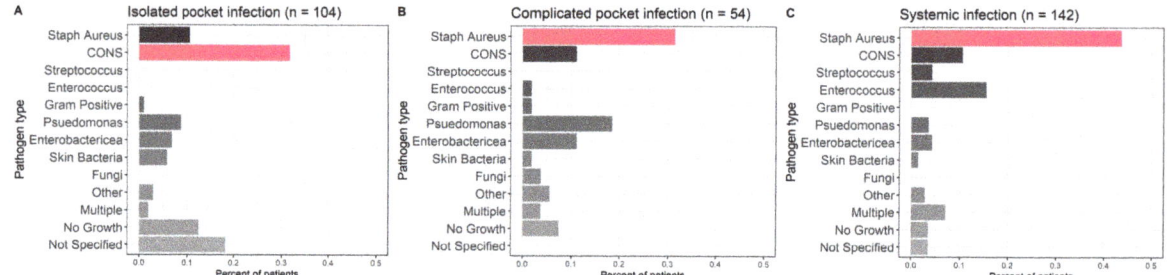

Figure 1. Infectious pathogens. *Staphylococcus aureus* was the most common pathogen responsible for CIED infection in the systemic (**C**) and complicated pocket infection (**B**) groups, while CONS was more frequent in the isolated pocket infection group (**A**).

3.2. Outcomes

3.2.1. Procedural Outcomes

A higher number of previous entries to the pocket were performed in the isolated and complicated pocket infection groups compared to the systemic infection group (2.4 ± 1.2 in the isolated and 2.2 ± 1.2 in the complicated pocket groups vs. 1.6 ± 0.9 in the systemic infection group, $p < 0.001$), with a temporal correlation from the last intervention to extraction (Table 3).

Complete removal of all leads (including tips) was achieved in 274/300 (91.3%) of the patients. In 18 patients (6%), partial removal was achieved, and in 6 patients (2%) the procedure was concluded as a failure (Table 3). Procedural success rates were achieved regardless of the etiology of extraction ($p = 0.724$) (Table 3). Complex tools were needed in most cases (69.7%), irrespective of the infection type ($p = 0.078$).

Major complications occurred in 7 (2.3%) patients and minor complications in 11 (3.7%) patients. Complication rates did not differ between groups (Table 3). Two patients died during the procedure and were excluded from further mortality analysis (one from each pocket infection group).

Table 3. Procedural details.

Infection Type	Overall	Pocket Isolated	Pocket Complicated	Systemic	p Value
Number of patients	300	104	54	142	
First device to extraction (days)	2691.7 ± 2187.3	2966.6 ± 2417.3	2814.0 ± 2003.0	2442.9 ± 2058.2	0.163
Current device to extraction (days)	1394.7 ± 1485.7	1170.1 ± 1304.9	1293.9 ± 1527.0	1600.9 ± 1576.6	0.076
Last intervention to extraction (days)	907.3 ± 975.1	705.5 ± 842.1	521.2 ± 684.3	1183.8 ± 1068.3	<0.001
Entries to pocket	2.0 (1.1)	2.4 (1.2)	2.2 (1.2)	1.6 (0.9)	<0.001
Extraction type					0.078
Simple	88 (29.3)	31 (29.8)	9 (16.7)	48 (33.8)	
Complex	209 (69.7)	73 (70.2)	43 (79.6)	93 (65.5)	
Unspecified	3 (1.0)	0 (0.0)	2 (3.7)	1 (0.7)	
Number of leads extracted	2.2 (0.9)	2.3 (0.9)	2.4 (1.0)	2.2 (0.8)	0.314
Extraction success					0.724
Full	274 (91.3)	94 (90.4)	49 (90.7)	131 (92.3)	
Partial	18 (6.0)	8 (7.7)	2 (3.7)	8 (5.6)	
Failure	6 (2.0)	2 (1.9)	2 (3.7)	2 (1.4)	
Unspecified	2 (0.7)	0 (0.0)	1 (1.9)	1 (0.7)	
Minor complications	11 (3.7)	4 (3.8)	2 (3.7)	5 (3.5)	0.991
Major complications	7 (2.3)	3 (2.9)	2 (3.7)	2 (1.4)	0.572
Temporary reimplant	77 (25.7)	27 (26.0)	19 (35.2)	31 (21.8)	0.160
Intra-procedural death	2 (0.7)	1 (1.0)	1 (1.9)	0 (0.0)	0.327

3.2.2. Reinfection Outcomes

Reinfection at 30 days was almost exclusive to the systemic infection group (n = 9, 6.3%, vs. one patient from each pocket infection group (p = 0.108)) (Table 4), even though patients in the pocket infection groups were reimplanted with a permanent device more often than the systemic infection group (80.8% isolated and 90.7% complicated vs. 68.3% for the systemic group, p = 0.002) (Table 4).

Table 4. Reinfection outcomes.

Infection Type	Overall	Pocket Isolated	Pocket Complicated	Systemic	p Value
Number of patients	300	104	54	142	
Permanent reimplant	230 (76.7)	84 (80.8)	49 (90.7)	97 (68.3)	0.002
Time to reimplant (days)	46 ± 103	53 ± 111	55 ± 78	34 ± 106	0.557
Infection within 30 days					0.108
No	134 (44.7)	53 (51.0)	25 (46.3)	56 (39.4)	
Yes	11 (3.7)	1 (1.0)	1 (1.9)	9 (6.3)	
Unspecified	155 (51.7)	50 (48.1)	28 (51.9)	77 (54.2)	

3.2.3. Mortality

During 30 days after the procedure, 33 patients (11%) died, and at the 1-year follow-up, 71 (23.7%) patients had died. Kaplan–Meier survival analysis (Figure 2) showed that at 3 years of follow-up, the rate of all-cause mortality was significantly higher among patients with systemic infections compared to both pocket infection groups (p < 0.001), with the curves diverging at 30 days. All-cause mortality was similar between both pocket infection groups, regardless of if they had vegetations or positive cultures (Supplementary Table S1).

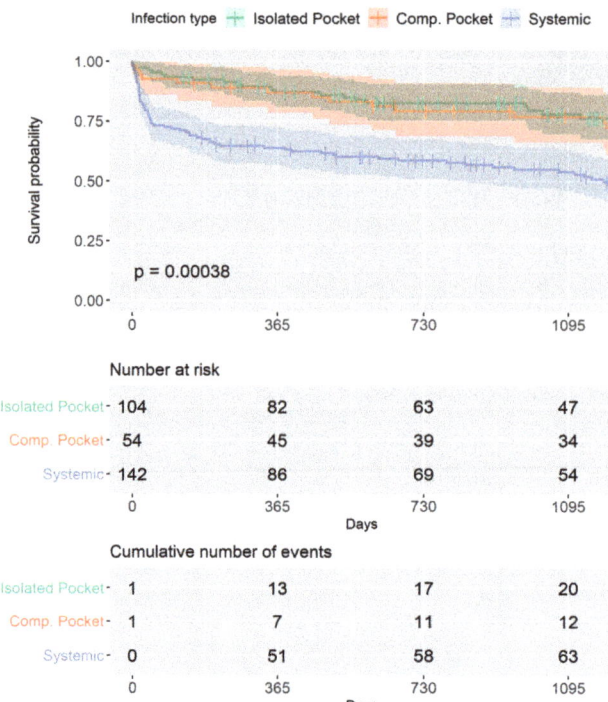

Figure 2. Overall survival for the entire study group. Kaplan–Meier survival analysis curves for each group. At 3 years of follow-up, the rate of all-cause mortality was significantly higher among patients with systemic infections compared to both pocket infection groups ($p < 0.001$), with the curves diverging at 30 days. All-cause mortality was similar between both pocket infection groups.

The univariate analysis showed that infection type, diabetes, lower hemoglobin, higher creatinine, leukocytosis, high temperature, lower albumin, and SA infection were all associated with short- and long-term mortality (Supplementary Table S2). Age, atrial fibrillation, heart failure, and vascular disease were found to predict long-term but not short-term mortality (Supplementary Table S3).

Multivariate analysis demonstrated that high creatinine and lower albumin were predictors of 30-day and 1-year mortality, while age and the presence of atrial fibrillation were predictors of 1-year mortality only (Table 5).

Table 5. Multivariate models for the prediction of mortality.

Mortality at 30 days	Odds ratio	Lower CI 95%	Upper CI 95%	p value
		At 30 days		
Diabetes mellitus	1.14	0.5	2.61	0.748
Creatinine (mg/dL)	1.43	1.03	1.99	0.034
Albumin (g/dL)	0.44	0.2	0.96	0.038
Hemoglobin (g/dL)	1.01	0.75	1.35	0.973
Lekuocytosis > 10K	1.43	0.63	3.25	0.392
Temperature > 37.8	0.79	0.29	2.17	0.654
Staph aureus	1.46	0.62	3.39	0.384
Isolated pocket infection	0.54	0.1	2.87	0.471
Systemic infection	1.43	0.42	4.89	0.557
		At 1 year		
Mortality at 1 year	Odds ratio	Lower CI 95%	Upper CI 95%	p value
Age	1.04	1	1.07	0.017
Atrial fibrillation	2.35	1.22	4.55	0.01
Heart failure	1.36	0.68	2.73	0.386
Vascular disease	1.11	0.53	2.29	0.785
Diabetes mellitus	1.04	0.52	2.09	0.905
Creatinine (mg/dL)	1.69	1.21	2.35	0.001
Albumin (g/dL)	0.33	0.17	0.64	< 0.001
Hemoglobin (g/dL)	1.12	0.88	1.43	0.339
Lekuocytosis > 10K	1.2	0.61	2.36	0.597
Temperature > 37.8	0.52	0.22	1.23	0.13
Staph aureus	1.34	0.64	2.8	0.433
Isolated pocket infection	1.06	0.32	3.48	0.925
Systemic infection	2.24	0.8	6.23	0.113

4. Discussion

Traditionally, patients rereferred for extraction were divided into pocket vs. systemic infection. This study characterized, for the first time, patients with complicated pocket infection, who differ from isolated pocket infection or systemic infection patients presenting for TLE. Most notably, these patients have special characteristics in the severity of their clinical presentation and microbiological pathogens; however, their outcome is significantly better than systemic infection and resembles those patients with isolated pocket infection.

CIED infections are usually categorized as either local pocket or endovascular, without differentiating the group of patients with positive BSI or vegetations secondary to generator pocket infection [16].

The present study distinguished between the two types of endovascular infections based on the involvement of the pocket site. This differentiation is important since the patients in each group have special characteristics and need different types of empiric therapy and treatment duration.

4.1. Patient Characteristics

The present study observed significant clinical differences between systemic and pocket infections. Diabetes seemed to be a risk factor for developing a systemic infection. In a previous meta-analysis, diabetes had an OR of 2.08 (1.62–2.67) for predicting CIED infection [17]; however, the meta-analysis did not distinguish the type of infection.

4.2. Infection Manifestation

Patients with a systemic infection had worse lab results, specifically those predicting a worse outcome, as described earlier by our group [18]. As expected, the lab results of the isolated pocket infection group were near normal, and those of the complicated pocket infection group were just in between the isolated and systemic groups.

Patients with complicated pocket infections had lower rates of fever and leukocytosis compared to those with systemic infections, perhaps suggesting that their diagnosis was earlier due to the local clinical signs and symptoms of pocket infection, while symptoms consistent with endocarditis resulted in a delayed diagnosis [11]. The complicated pocket infection group was treated as the systemic infection group, which was significantly longer than the isolated pocket infection group.

Although positive pocket cultures were obtained in majority of both pocket infection groups, a small percentage of the systemic group had positive pocket cultures as well, perhaps secondary to direct contamination of extracting infected leads through the pocket.

Blood cultures were positive in 83.8% and 53.7% of patients in the systemic only group and the complicated pocket group, respectively. This may also explain the better prognosis of the latter group and reflect the different pathogenesis of infection between the two groups.

Interestingly, the lead culture was positive in a similar percentage of all patients. TTE and TEE observed vegetations in a similar percentage of patients in the complicated pocket and systemic infection groups, probably related to SA, the major pathogen of these groups, as opposed to the higher CONS infection in the isolated pocket group (Figure 1). These results are in accordance with previous studies that compared systemic vs. pocket infections [19–22]. As was shown before [23], both pocket infection groups had a high percentage of Gram-negative bacteria in comparison to the systemic group.

4.3. Outcomes

Complete removal of all leads was achieved in most of our cohort (91%), with no difference in the tools used for the extraction procedure or complication rates between the groups. There were more entries to the pocket with a shorter time passing from the last intervention to infection manifestation for both pocket infection groups, signifying the casual relation between entering the pocket and its infection. This observation has been previously recognized and explained by repeated extractions and reimplantation, which could cause an inflammation and repeated bacterial colonization, leading to an infection [19].

In our study, 76.7% of patients were reimplanted with a permanent device within 46 ± 103 days, with 3.7% of the cohort suffering from reinfection during the first 30 days. These numbers are slightly higher than a previous study from the United States (1.3%) [24]. An intriguing finding of our study was the reinfection rate of 6.3% at 30 days for the systemic infection group, as opposed to that in each of the pocket infection groups, even though the latter groups were implanted more often with a permanent device after the procedure ($p = 0.002$). These findings deserve further attention in future studies in order to find which criteria are needed in choosing the patients for implantation of a CIED after undergoing a TLE. Other inflammatory markers, such as C-reactive protein and procalcitonin, could play a role in predicting the severity and type of the CIED infection. These parameters were not included in this analysis due to a lack of data.

4.4. Mortality

Mortality in our cohort was similar to that previously reported at one year (23.7%) [25,26]. An important observation is the worse outcome for the systemic group after three years of follow-up, with significantly higher mortality rates among patients with systemic infections compared to pocket infections, as was reported by the ELECTRA study [26], without a difference whether the pocket infection was complicated or not. Interestingly, our study showed, for the first time, a diversion in the Kaplan–Meier curves after 30 days post-TLE, as opposed to previous studies where no difference could be found in the mortality rates between groups after 12 months [27,28]. More significant is our finding of similar outcomes for each pocket infection group (complicated and isolated), implying that even though there are many similarities between the systemic infection and complicated pocket infection (hematogenous spread of infection resulting in infective endocarditis), these are different prognostic groups, which should be regarded as such. These findings are in contrast to a previous publication, where the type of CIED infection presentation was also a strong predictor for one-year mortality in patients with pocket infection who had positive blood cultures or vegetation on the leads (similar to our complicated pocket infection group), who had a one-year mortality that was higher than patients with pocket infection with negative blood cultures and no vegetation [25].

5. Conclusions

Patients with CIED infection due to a complicated pocket infection present with clinical characteristics of systemic infection that are milder than patients with endovascular infection alone. The most prevalent microbiological pathogen is SA; however, they have a high rate of Gram-negative bacteria as well. Despite the systemic pattern of the infection, their prognosis is similar to the isolated pocket infection group, and this might be due to the earlier diagnosis, wider range of causative pathogens, and lower rates of BSI. We suggest that this special category be presented separately in future publications of CIED infections. It is important to differentiate between all infection groups to provide the best treatment option and timing of CIED reimplantation.

6. Limitations

The main limitation of this study is that it was a retrospective analysis of a single center. Another limiting factor is that not all patients completed their follow-up, mainly those that were referred from other hospitals.

Supplementary Materials: The following supporting information can be downloaded at: https://www.mdpi.com/article/10.3390/jcm12134397/s1, Table S1. The different mortality rates between groups at different time points. Table S2: Univariate analysis of 30-day mortality. Table S3. Univariate analysis of one-year mortality.

Author Contributions: Conceptualization, E.N. and A.W.-F.; methodology, E.N., A.M. (Anat Milman), and A.W.-F.; software, G.Z.; validation, E.N., A.M. (Anat Milman) and A.W.-F.; formal analysis, G.Z. and A.M. (Anat Milman); investigation, A.M. (Amit Meitus), S.K. and Y.S.; data curation, A.M. (Anat Milman); writing—original draft preparation, A.M. (Anat Milman); writing—review and editing, E.N., R.B., A.W.-F. and G.R.; visualization, A.M. (Anat Milman); supervision, E.N. and A.W.-F.; project administration, A.M. (Anat Milman). All authors have read and agreed to the published version of the manuscript.

Funding: This research received no external funding.

Institutional Review Board Statement: The study was conducted according to the guidelines of the Declaration of Helsinki and approved by the Institutional Review Board of Sheba Medical Center.

Informed Consent Statement: Informed consent was obtained from all subjects involved in the study.

Data Availability Statement: The data presented in this study are available upon request from the corresponding author.

Conflicts of Interest: The authors declare no conflict of interest.

References

1. Brignole, M.; Auricchio, A.; Baron-Esquivias, G.; Bordachar, P.; Boriani, G.; Breithardt, O.A.; Cleland, J.G.F.; Deharo, J.-C.; Delgado, V.; Elliott, P.M.; et al. 2013 ESC guidelines on cardiac pacing and cardiac resynchronization therapy: The task force on cardiac pacing and resynchronization therapy of the European Society of Cardiology (ESC). Developed in collaboration with the European Heart Rhythm Association (EHRA). *Europace* **2013**, *15*, 1070–1118. [PubMed]
2. Epstein, A.E.; Dimarco, J.P.; Ellenbogen, K.A.; Estes, N.A., 3rd; Freedman, R.A.; Gettes, L.S.; American College of Cardiology/American Heart Association Task Force on Practice; American Association for Thoracic Surgery; Society of Thoracic Surgeons. ACC/AHA/HRS 2008 guidelines for Device-Based Therapy of Cardiac Rhythm Abnormalities: Executive summary. *Heart Rhythm* **2008**, *5*, 934–955. [CrossRef] [PubMed]

3. Wilkoff, B.L.; Love, C.J.; Byrd, C.L.; Bongiorni, M.G.; Carrillo, R.G.; Crossley, G.H., 3rd; Epstein, L.M.; Friedman, R.A.; Kennergren, C.E.; Mitkowski, P.; et al. Transvenous lead extraction: Heart Rhythm Society expert consensus on facilities, training, indications, and patient man-agement: This document was endorsed by the American Heart Association (AHA). *Heart Rhythm* **2009**, *6*, 1085–1104. [CrossRef] [PubMed]
4. Baddour, L.M.; Epstein, A.E.; Erickson, C.C.; Knight, B.P.; Levison, M.E.; Lockhart, P.B.; Masoudi, F.A.; Okum, E.J.; Wilson, W.R.; Beerman, L.B.; et al. Update on cardiovascular implantable electronic device infections and their management: A scientific statement from the American Heart Association. *Circulation* **2010**, *121*, 458–477. [CrossRef] [PubMed]
5. Maytin, M.; Epstein, L.M. The challenges of transvenous lead extraction. *Heart* **2011**, *97*, 425–434. [CrossRef]
6. Deharo, J.C.; Bongiorni, M.G.; Rozkovec, A.; Bracke, F.; Defaye, P.; Fernandez-Lozano, I.; Golzio, P.G.; Hansky, B.; Kennergren, C.; Manolis, A.; et al. Pathways for training and accreditation for transvenous lead extraction: A European Heart Rhythm Association position paper. *Europace* **2012**, *14*, 124–134.
7. Sohal, M.; Williams, S.E.; Arujuna, A.; Chen, Z.; Bostock, J.; Gill, J.S.; Rinaldi, C.A. The current practice and perception of cardiac implantable electronic device transvenous lead extraction in the UK. *Europace* **2013**, *15*, 865–870. [CrossRef]
8. Blomström-Lundqvist, C.; Traykov, V.; Erba, P.A.; Burri, H.; Nielsen, J.C.; Bongiorni, M.G.; Poole, J.; Boriani, G.; Costa, R.; Deharo, J.C.; et al. European Heart Rhythm Association (EHRA) international consensus document on how to prevent, diagnose, and treat cardiac implantable electronic device infections-endorsed by the Heart Rhythm Society (HRS), the Asia Pacific Heart Rhythm Society (APHRS), the Latin American Heart Rhythm Society (LAHRS), International Society for Cardiovascular Infectious Diseases (ISCVID), and the European Society of Clinical Microbiology and Infectious Diseases (ESCMID) in collaboration with the European Association for Cardio-Thoracic Surgery (EACTS). *Eur. Heart J.* **2020**, *41*, 2012–2032.
9. Kleemann, T.; Becker, T.; Strauss, M.; Dyck, N.; Weisse, U.; Saggau, W.; Burkhardt, U.; Seidl, K. Prevalence of bacterial colonization of generator pockets in implantable cardioverter defibrillator patients without signs of infection undergoing generator replacement or lead revision. *Europace* **2010**, *12*, 58–63. [CrossRef]
10. Chambers, S.T. Diagnosis and management of staphylococcal infections of pacemakers and cardiac defibrillators. *Intern. Med. J.* **2005**, *35* (Suppl. 2), S63–S71. [CrossRef]
11. Klug, D.; Lacroix, D.; Savoye, C.; Goullard, L.; Grandmougin, D.; Hennequin, J.L.; Kacet, S.; Lekieffre, J. Systemic infection related to endocarditis on pacemaker leads: Clinical presentation and management. *Circulation* **1997**, *95*, 2098–2107. [CrossRef]
12. Hussein, A.A.; Baghdy, Y.; Wazni, O.M.; Brunner, M.P.; Kabbach, G.; Shao, M.; Gordon, S.; Saliba, W.I.; Wilkoff, B.L.; Tarakji, K.G. Microbiology of cardiac implantable electronic device infections. *JACC Clin. Electrophysiol.* **2016**, *2*, 498–505. [CrossRef]
13. Bongiorni, M.G.; Tascini, C.; Tagliaferri, E.; Di Cori, A.; Soldati, E.; Leonildi, A.; Zucchelli, G.; Ciullo, I.; Menichetti, F. Microbiology of cardiac implantable electronic device infections. *Europace* **2012**, *14*, 1334–1339. [CrossRef]
14. Younis, A.; Glikson, M.; Meitus, A.; Arwas, N.; Natanzon, S.S.; Lotan, D.; Luria, D.; Beinart, R.; Nof, E. Transvenous lead extraction with laser reduces need for femoral approach during the procedure. *PLoS ONE* **2019**, *14*, e0215589. [CrossRef]
15. Sandoe, J.A.; Barlow, G.; Chambers, J.B.; Gammage, M.; Guleri, A.; Howard, P.; Olson, E.; Perry, J.D.; Prendergast, B.D.; Spry, M.J.; et al. Guidelines for the diagnosis, prevention and management of implantable cardiac electronic device infection. Report of a joint Working Party project on behalf of the British Society for Antimicrobial Chemotherapy (BSAC, host organization), British Heart Rhythm Society (BHRS), British Cardiovascular Society (BCS), British Heart Valve Society (BHVS) and British Society for Echocardiography (BSE). *J. Antimicrob. Chemother.* **2015**, *70*, 325–359.
16. Tarakji, K.G.; Chan, E.J.; Cantillon, D.J.; Doonan, A.L.; Hu, T.; Schmitt, S.; Fraser, T.G.; Kim, A.; Gordon, S.M.; Wilkoff, B.L. Cardiac implantable electronic device infections: Presentation, management, and patient outcomes. *Heart Rhythm* **2010**, *7*, 1043–1047. [CrossRef] [PubMed]
17. Polyzos, K.A.; Konstantelias, A.A.; Falagas, M.E. Risk factors for cardiac implantable electronic device infection: A systematic review and meta-analysis. *Europace* **2015**, *17*, 767–777. [CrossRef]
18. Milman, A.; Zahavi, G.; Meitus, A.; Kariv, S.; Shafir, Y.; Glikson, M.; Luria, D.; Beinart, R.; Nof, E. Predictors of short-term mortality in patients undergoing a successful uncomplicated extraction procedure. *J. Cardiovasc. Electrophysiol.* **2020**, *31*, 1155–1162. [CrossRef]
19. Hörnsten, J.; Axelsson, L.; Westling, K. Cardiac Implantable Electronic Device Infections: Long-Term Outcome after Extraction and Antibiotic Treatment. *Infect. Dis. Rep.* **2021**, *13*, 59. [CrossRef]
20. Uslan, D.Z.; Sohail, M.R.; St Sauver, J.L.; Friedman, P.A.; Hayes, D.L.; Stoner, S.M.; Wilson, W.R.; Steckelberg, J.M.; Baddour, L.M. Permanent pacemaker and implantable cardioverter defibrillator infection: A population-based study. *Arch. Intern. Med.* **2007**, *167*, 669–675. [CrossRef]
21. Fukunaga, M.; Goya, M.; Nagashima, M.; Hiroshima, K.; Yamada, T.; An, Y.; Hayashi, K.; Makihara, Y.; Ohe, M.; Ichihashi, K.; et al. Identification of causative organism in cardiac implantable electronic device infections. *J. Cardiol.* **2017**, *70*, 411–415. [CrossRef] [PubMed]
22. Carrasco, F.; Anguita, M.; Ruiz, M.; Castillo, J.C.; Delgado, M.; Mesa, D.; Romo, E.; Pan, M.; De Lezo, J.S. Clinical features and changes in epidemiology of infective endocarditis on pacemaker devices over a 27-year period (1987–2013). *Europace* **2016**, *18*, 836–841. [CrossRef] [PubMed]

23. Esquer Garrigos, Z.; George, M.P.; Vijayvargiya, P.; Tan, E.M.; Farid, S.; Abu Saleh, O.M.; Friedman, P.A.; Steckelberg, J.M.; DeSimone, D.C.; Wilson, W.R.; et al. Clinical Presentation, Management, and Outcomes of Cardiovascular Implantable Electronic Device Infections Due to Gram-Negative Versus Gram-Positive Bacteria. *Mayo Clin. Proc.* **2019**, *94*, 1268–1277. [CrossRef] [PubMed]
24. Boyle, T.A.; Uslan, D.Z.; Prutkin, J.M.; Greenspon, A.J.; Baddour, L.M.; Danik, S.B.; Tolosana, J.M.; Le, K.; Miro, J.M.; Peacock, J.; et al. Reimplantation and Repeat Infection After Cardiac-Implantable Electronic Device Infections: Experience from the MEDIC (Multicenter Electrophysiologic Device Infection Cohort) Database. *Circ. Arrhythm. Electrophysiol.* **2017**, *10*, e004822. [CrossRef]
25. Tarakji, K.G.; Wazni, O.M.; Harb, S.; Hsu, A.; Saliba, W.; Wilkoff, B.L. Risk factors for 1-year mortality among patients with cardiac implantable electronic device infection undergoing transvenous lead extraction: The impact of the infection type and the presence of vegetation on survival. *Europace* **2014**, *16*, 1490–1495. [CrossRef]
26. Bongiorni, M.G.; Kennergren, C.; Butter, C.; Deharo, J.C.; Kutarski, A.; Rinaldi, C.A.; Romano, S.L.; Maggioni, A.P.; Andarala, M.; Auricchio, A.; et al. The European Lead Extraction ConTRolled (ELECTRa) study: A European Heart Rhythm Association (EHRA) Registry of Transvenous Lead Extraction Outcomes. *Eur. Heart J.* **2017**, *38*, 2995–3005. [CrossRef]
27. Nishii, N.; Morimoto, Y.; Miyoshi, A.; Tsukuda, S.; Miyamoto, M.; Kawada, S.; Nakagawa, K.; Watanabe, A.; Nakamura, K.; Morita, H.; et al. Prognosis after lead extraction in patients with cardiac implantable electronic devices infection: Comparison of lead-related infective endocarditis with pocket infection in a Japanese single-center experience. *J. Arrhythm.* **2019**, *35*, 654–663. [CrossRef]
28. Ihlemann, N.; Møller-Hansen, M.; Salado-Rasmussen, K.; Videbæk, R.; Moser, C.; Iversen, K.; Bundgaard, H. CIED infection with either pocket or systemic infection presentation—Complete device removal and long-term antibiotic treatment; long-term outcome. *Scand. Cardiovasc. J.* **2016**, *50*, 52–57. [CrossRef]

Disclaimer/Publisher's Note: The statements, opinions and data contained in all publications are solely those of the individual author(s) and contributor(s) and not of MDPI and/or the editor(s). MDPI and/or the editor(s) disclaim responsibility for any injury to people or property resulting from any ideas, methods, instructions or products referred to in the content.

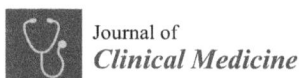 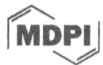

Article

Identification of Pacemaker Lead Position Using Fluoroscopy to Avoid Significant Tricuspid Regurgitation

Dicky A. Hanafy [1], Amiliana M. Soesanto [1], Budhi Setianto [1], Suzanna Immanuel [2], Sunu B. Raharjo [1], Herqutanto [3], Muzakkir Amir [4] and Yoga Yuniadi [1,*]

[1] Department of Cardiology and Vascular Medicine, Faculty of Medicine, Universitas Indonesia, National Cardiovascular Center Harapan Kita, Jakarta 11420, Indonesia; drdhanafy@yahoo.de (D.A.H.); amiliana14@gmail.com (A.M.S.); heybudhi@gmail.com (B.S.); sunu.b.raharjo@gmail.com (S.B.R.)
[2] Department of Clinical Pathology, Faculty of Medicine, Universitas Indonesia, Dr. Cipto Mangunkusumo National Central Public Hospital, Jakarta 10430, Indonesia; suzanna.immanuel@gmail.com
[3] Department of Community Medicine, Faculty of Medicine, Universitas Indonesia, Jakarta 12345, Indonesia; hqtanto@gmail.com
[4] Department of Cardiology and Vascular Medicine, Faculty of Medicine, Universitas Hasanuddin, Dr. Wahidin Sudirohusodo Cardiovascular Center, Makassar 90245, Indonesia; dr.muzakkir@gmail.com
* Correspondence: yogay136@gmail.com; Tel.: +62-8111277889

Abstract: Permanent pacemaker implantation improves survival but can cause tricuspid valve dysfunction in the form of tricuspid regurgitation (TR). The dominant mechanism of pacemaker-mediated TR is lead impingement. This study evaluated the association between the location of the pacemaker leads crossing the tricuspid valve and the incidence of worsening TR and lead impingement using fluoroscopy. Lead positions were evaluated using perpendicular right anterior oblique (RAO) and parallel left anterior oblique (LAO) fluoroscopic angulation views of the tricuspid annulus. A two-dimensional transthoracic echocardiogram (TTE) was performed to evaluate the maximum TR jet area-to-right atrium ratio and define regurgitation severity. A three-dimensional TTE was performed to evaluate lead impingement. A worsening of TR was observed in 23 of 82 subjects. Most leads had an inferior position in the RAO view and a septal position in the LAO view. The mid position in the RAO view and septal position in the LAO view were risk factors for lead impingement. Mid and septal positions were associated with higher risks of significant TR and lead impingement. Lead impingement was associated with a high risk of significant TR. Pacemaker-mediated TR remains a significant problem after lead implantation.

Keywords: fluoroscopy; jet area; lead impingement; transthoracic echocardiogram; tricuspid regurgitation

1. Introduction

Permanent pacemaker (PPM) implantation is associated with undesirable effects on the tricuspid valve structure and function. Structural effects include valve damage during lead placement, mechanical interruption of normal leaflet coaptation, leaflet entrapment, entanglement of the subvalvular support structure, and endocarditis [1]. Functional effects include valvular stenosis and tricuspid valve regurgitation (TR). The right ventricle pacemaker lead crossing the tricuspid valve may cause fibrosis and thickening of the leaflets, thus impairing valve mobility and coaptation. Current pacemaker lead implantation procedures are guided by fluoroscopy and do not allow an evaluation of the tricuspid valve structure or function after the intracardiac leads have been implanted.

Moderate and severe TR based on echocardiography findings are classified as significant TR [2]. PPM implantation with the use of an RV lead crossing the tricuspid valve is associated with a two-fold higher risk of significant TR [3]. Pacemaker-mediated TR (PMTR) occurs when the pacemaker leads cause damage to the valve leaflets. It can also occur secondary due to RV dilatation and dysfunction caused by chronic dyssynchronous

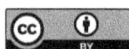

Citation: Hanafy, D.A.; Soesanto, A.M.; Setianto, B.; Immanuel, S.; Raharjo, S.B.; Herqutanto; Amir, M.; Yuniadi, Y. Identification of Pacemaker Lead Position Using Fluoroscopy to Avoid Significant Tricuspid Regurgitation. *J. Clin. Med.* **2023**, *12*, 4782. https://doi.org/10.3390/jcm12144782

Academic Editors: Ibrahim Marai and Urs Eriksson

Received: 26 April 2023
Revised: 7 June 2023
Accepted: 17 July 2023
Published: 19 July 2023

Copyright: © 2023 by the authors. Licensee MDPI, Basel, Switzerland. This article is an open access article distributed under the terms and conditions of the Creative Commons Attribution (CC BY) license (https://creativecommons.org/licenses/by/4.0/).

RV pacing [4]. A previous observational study showed that TR occurred when implanted device leads interfered with the normal tricuspid valve leaflet motion as viewed during a three-dimensional (3D) transthoracic echocardiogram (TTE); however, an association between the device lead position and TR incidence was not observed [5]. Another study noted that pacemaker lead positions on the annulus or inter-leaflet cleft that interfere with valvular mechanics can result in PMTR [3]. The position of pacemaker leads in the tricuspid valve can be identified using fluoroscopy, echocardiography, computed tomography, and magnetic resonance imaging.

The mechanisms of pacemaker-mediated TR are relatively unknown. They may include mechanical interference with tricuspid valve movement resulting in impingement, fibrosis, and excessive scarring. Inflammation and tissue fibrosis as well as scar formation involving valve tissues have been reported with PMTR [6,7].

Lin et al. reported that pacemaker lead impingement caused TR in 39% of 41 subjects; however, it was not associated with PPM lead positions [8]. Because PMTR is largely asymptomatic initially, its prevalence and relationship with PPM lead positions are understudied. Our study aimed to identify the positions of the pacemaker lead that are associated with significant TR.

2. Materials and Methods

This retrospective cohort study was conducted at the Harapan Kita National Cardiovascular Centre in Jakarta, Indonesia, from June 2020 to April 2021. The study population consisted of patients who underwent PPM implantation and were recruited consecutively from the medical record database and provided informed consent. Patients' echocardiography was assessed at baseline and after implantation. Patients underwent noninvasive fluoroscopy assessment of pacemaker lead position. Inclusion criteria were as follows: age older than 18 years; underwent routine follow-up after PPM implantation; willing to participate in the study; and no previous right ventricular dysfunction (tricuspid annular plane systolic excursion [TAPSE] > 1.6 cm). The exclusion criteria were as follows: congenital or primary tricuspid disorder; left cardiac dysfunction with ejection fraction < 35%; pulmonary hypertension as defined by ESC/ERS Guidelines [9]; body constitution complicating echocardiography; more than one lead crossing the tricuspid valve; and rheumatic heart disease. This study did not include patients with permanent pacemakers with a single atrial lead, implantable cardioverter defibrillators (ICDs), or cardiac resynchronization therapy (CRT) devices. Information on patient comorbidities (coronary heart disease, hypertension, diabetes mellitus, atrial fibrillation) was acquired from the electronic medical record. Patients with heart failure included those with reduced or preserved ejection fraction. The study was approved by the Medical Research Ethic Committee of Universitas Indonesia Medical School in Jakarta, Indonesia. We did not conduct any special intervention or experiment; subjects underwent a non-invasive fluoroscopy examination and transthoracic echocardiography.

2.1. Fluoroscopy

Fluoroscopy angulation was performed to obtain en face and perpendicular in-plane views to evaluate the position of the pacemaker lead crossing the tricuspid valve annulus. Evaluation of the pacemaker lead position was viewed using the right anterior oblique (RAO) and left anterior oblique (LAO) projections. In the RAO position, the C-arm was angulated 30°; then, the annulus, which was seen as more radiolucent than the surrounding area, was evaluated. The radiolucent part was expected to be perpendicular when adjusting the RAO angulation by 30° to 40°, and the thinnest part was considered the most perpendicular annulus. We recorded the 3 s or three-heartbeat motion image (cineangiography) with RAO angulation. With LAO angulation, the C-arm was rotated 55° and 12° caudally to achieve a parallel en face tricuspid valve view; then, we recorded the 3 s or three-heartbeat motion image (cineangiography).

In the RAO view, the pacemaker lead position was categorized into three locations, superior (S) mid (M), and inferior (I), in the annulus radiolucent position. In the LAO view, the pacemaker lead position was classified as lateral (1) or septal (2) (Figure 1).

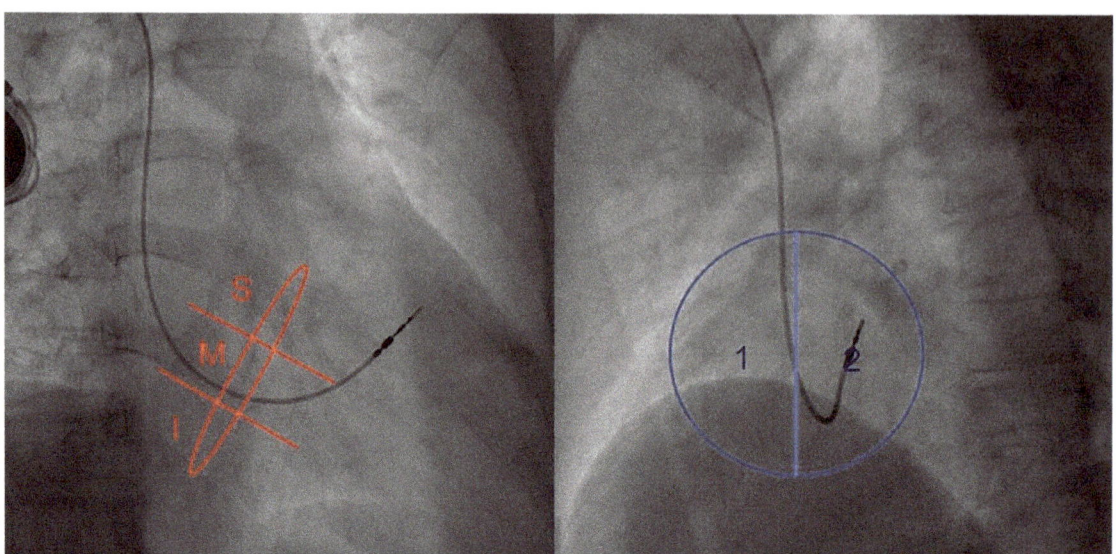

Figure 1. Mid-septal lead positions in the right anterior oblique (RAO) and left anterior oblique (LAO) views. S, superior; M, middle; I, inferior; 1, lateral position; 2, septal position.

2.2. Transthoracic Echocardiogram

Trans-thoracic echocardiography (TTE) was performed before and after pacemaker implantation. Two-dimensional and 3D TTEs were performed by independent echocardiographers using GE Vivid E9 (GE Vingmed Ultrasound AS, Horten, Norway), GE Vivid E95 (GE Vingmed Ultrasound AS, Horten, Norway), and Philips Epiq Cvx (Philips Ultrasound, Bothell, WA, USA) with standard views: parasternal long and sort axis, apical, and subcostal views with M-mode, 2-dimensional echocardiography, and color Doppler ultrasonography. Two-dimensional TTE measured echocardiographic standard parameters such as the left ventricular internal dimension in diastole, left ventricular internal dimension in systole, ejection fraction measured by the Simpsons method, right ventricle dimensions, left atrium dimensions, vena contracta (VC), and regurgitation severity by comparing the maximum TR jet area with the right atrium area. Tricuspid annular plane systolic excursion (TAPSE) was measured on M-mode recordings of the lateral tricuspid annulus in an RV-focused view. The severity of tricuspid regurgitation was graded on a 5-point scale; 0 = no, 1 = trace, 2 = mild, 3 = moderate, and 4 = severe. Significant TR was defined as: moderate to severe TR as defined by the recommended parameters of the American Society of Echocardiography, with jet area-to-right atrium ratio $\geq$ 20% and VC $\geq$ 0.3 cm [10]. TR was not significant if the TR jet area-to-right atrium ratio < 20% and VC < 0.3 cm or mild based on the recommended parameters of the American Society of Echocardiography guidelines (Figure 2) [10].

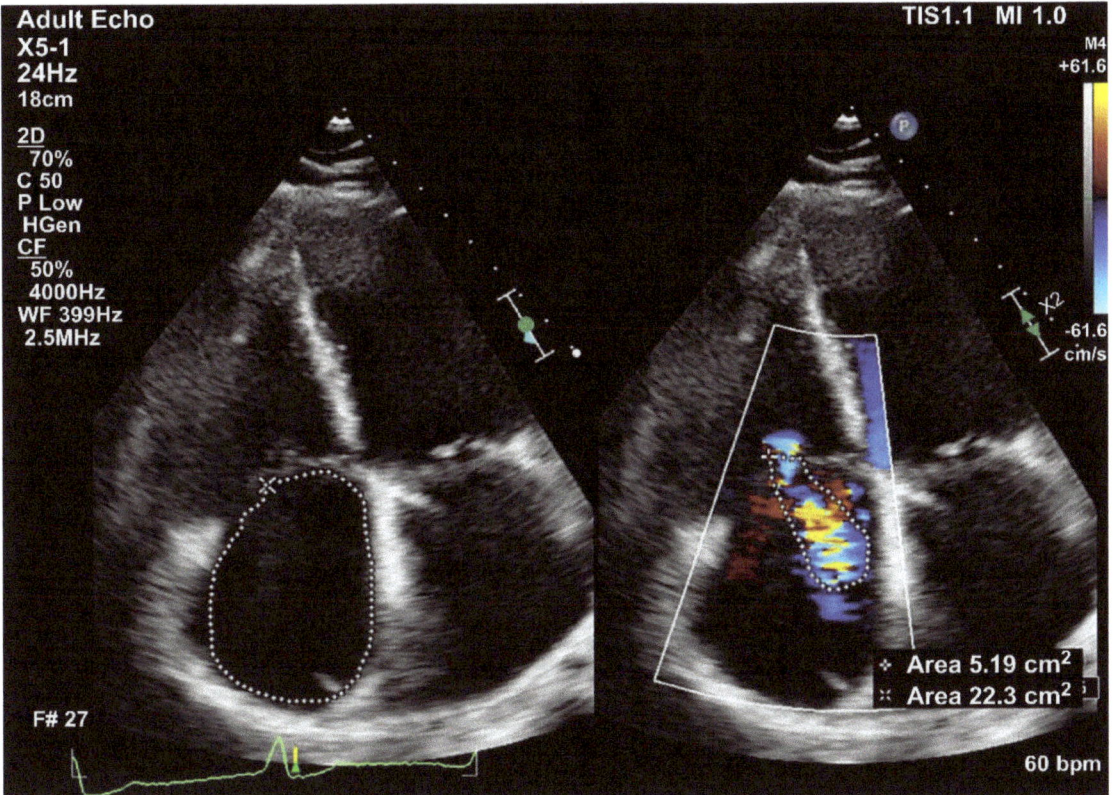

Figure 2. Tricuspid regurgitation (TR) jet area-to-right atrium ratio in the end-systolic phase measured using two-dimensional transthoracic echocardiography. The left panel shows the right atrium area (dot line = 22.3 cm²). The right panel shows the TR jet area (dot line = 5.19 cm²). The TR jet area-to-right atrium ratio = 23.3% (>20% is considered significant TR).

The 3D TTE was performed using the standard position and en face view. We evaluated the tricuspid valve morphology, pacemaker lead position, and lead impingement. Lead impingement on the anterior, posterior, and septal leaflets of the tricuspid valve was defined as impinging; however, a pacemaker lead located in the anteroposterior, anteroseptal, and posteroseptal commissures or with a central position (in the middle of coaptation and with no impingement on the tricuspid leaflet) was defined as non-impinging (Figure 3). The echocardiographer was blind to the fluoroscopy results of the lead position.

2.3. Study Variables

The dependent variables were the presence of worsening to significant TR as defined. Patients who had the same degree of TR (non-significant or significant TR) at baseline and did not progress to a worse degree of TR post-implantation were defined as non-worsening TR. The independent variables were the pacemaker lead position (evaluated by fluoroscopy) and lead impingement on the tricuspid valve (evaluated by 3D TTE).

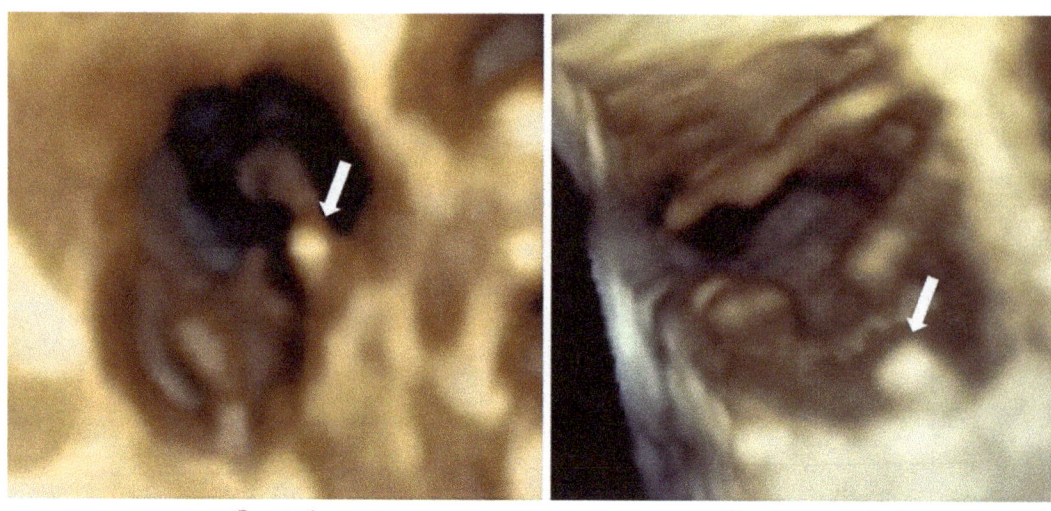

Septal   Posteroseptal

Figure 3. Pacemaker lead position viewed with three-dimensional (3D) transthoracic echocardiography. From left-to-right: (1) pacemaker lead observed as impinging on the septal leaflet; and (2) pacemaker lead observed in the posteroseptal commissure. Arrows point to the pacemaker lead.

2.4. Statistical Analysis

Data were expressed as mean ± standard deviation (if normally distributed) or median ± interquartile range (if not normally distributed). The normality of the distribution of variables was assessed using the Kolmogorov–Smirnov test. Associations between two categorical variables were evaluated using the chi-square test or Fisher's test. Mean differences between two groups were analyzed with the unpaired t-test (if normally distributed) or Mann–Whitney test (if not normally distributed). A two-tailed $p < 0.05$ was considered statistically significant. A multivariate analysis was performed for significant variables, and a logistic regression model was used to identify the risk factors for TR. Data were processed using SPSS version 25.0 software (IBM Corp., Armonk, NY, USA).

3. Results

The study included a final sample size of 80 subjects with a mean age of 61.3 ± 12.27 years; 58.5% females). During 2018 until the end of 2020, there were 799 patients who were implanted with a pacemaker (Figure 4) A significant number of patients with sinus node dysfunction were implanted with atrial single chamber pacemaker due to cost, which were excluded from this study. There was also a significant number of patients who did not have an echocardiogram before pacemaker implantation at our center but mostly at the referring centers without detailed description. Lastly, a significant number of patients had no follow up echo because these patients were referred back to the referring centers or refused to participate in the study. Hence no 3D echo could be performed mostly because of the distance to our center and the health referral system in our country.

The indications for pacemaker implantation were complete heart block (57.3%), sinus node dysfunction (29.3%), or other AV nodal conduction disturbance (13.4%). Other AV nodal conduction disturbances were defined as incomplete heart block either type 2 s degree AV block or trifascicular block. Most patients had a dual-chamber pacemaker (72.0%). The median pacing percentage was 100%. The patients had a mean implantation duration of 35.22 months (standard deviation 35.81 months). At baseline, non-significant TR was noted in 80 (95.6%) patients, and moderate to severe TR was noted in 2 (2.4%) patients. Of the patients with non-significant TR at baseline, the TR remained non-significant in 57 (71.25%)

patients at the time of the study. TR worsened to significant TR in 23 (26.25%) patients. In one patient, TR improved and became non-significant. Hence, worsening TR was present in a significant proportion of patients (Table 1). There were no differences in RA and RV dimensions, TAPSE, or RV fractional area change (FAC). The patients with worsening TR were, on average, older and had a longer mean duration of pacemaker implantation but these differences were not statistically significant. Age, sex, hypertension, coronary heart disease, atrial fibrillation, and heart failure were clinical factors associated with a worsening TR.

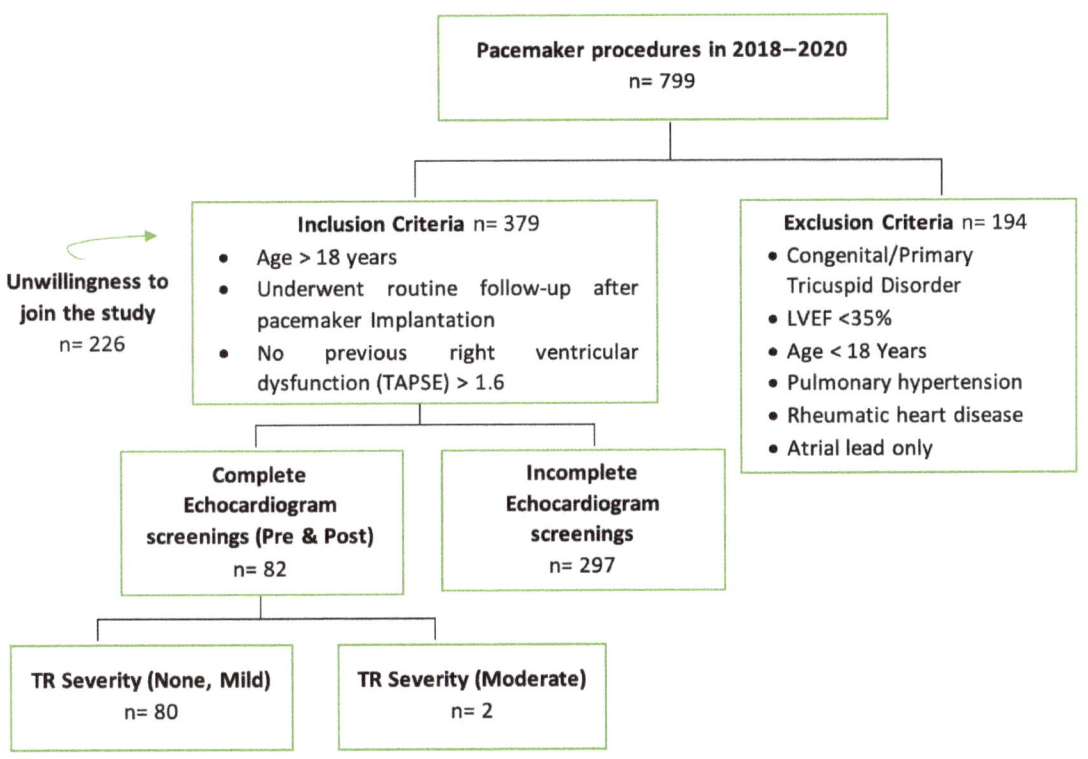

Figure 4. Flow diagram of patients receiving a pacemaker included in the study.

Table 1. Baseline characteristics.

Characteristics	Tricuspid Regurgitation		OR (95% CI)	p-Value
	Worsening TR (n = 23)	Not Worsening TR (n = 57)		
Sex, n (%)				
Male	7 (30.4)	25 (43.9)	0.56 (0.20–1.57)	0.267 *
Female	16 (69.6)	32 (56.1)		
Mean age, years	63.35 ± 11.24	59.93 ± 12.70		0.221 †
History of coronary heart disease				
Yes	9 (39.1)	11 (19.3)	2.69 (0.93–7.80)	0.064 *
No	14 (60.9)	46 (80.7)		
Hypertension				
Yes	20 (87.0)	35 (61.4)	4.19 (1.11–15.77)	0.026 *

Table 1. Cont.

Characteristics	Tricuspid Regurgitation		OR (95% CI)	p-Value
	Worsening TR (n = 23)	Not Worsening TR (n = 57)		
No	3 (13.0)	22 (38.6)		
Diabetes mellitus, type 2				
Yes	7 (30.4)	21 (35.6)	0.75 (0.27–2.12)	0.587 *
No	16 (69.6)	36 (63.2)		
Atrial fibrillation				
Yes	8 (34.8)	11 (19.3)	2.23 (0.76–6.58)	0.141 *
No	15 (65.2)	46 (80.7)		
History of heart failure				
Yes	10 (43.5)	14 (24.6)	2.36 (0.85–6.56)	0.095 *
No	13 (56.5)	43 (75.4)		
Mean PPM implantation duration, months/median	43.91 ± 40.52/32 (7–151)	32.51 ± 33.96/24 (8–179)		0.271 †
Median pacing percentage	100.0 (2.1–100.0)	100.0 (0.2–100.0)		0.591 †
PPM indication				
Sinus node dysfunction	7 (30.4)	16 (28.1)		0.706
Complete heart block	14 (60.9)	32 (56.1)		
Other AV conduction disturbance	2 (8.7)	9 (15.8)		
PPM type				
Single chamber	8 (34.8%)	14 (24.6%)	1.64 (0.57–4.67)	0.354 *
Dual chamber	15 (65.2%)	43 (75.4%)		
Echocardiography				
LVEF, %	61.86 ± 14.00	65.48 ± 10.87		0.257 ‡
LVIDd, mm	48.49 ± 5.80	47.05 ± 8.95		0.481 ‡
LVIDs, mm	30.46 ± 7.87	28.57 ± 7.86		0.395 †
LAVI, mL/mm^2	40.57 ± 17.13	36.12 ± 12.55		0.233 †
Left atrial dimension, mm	39.72 ± 7.03	37.90 ± 6.98		0.305 †
TAPSE, mm	21.67 ± 4.07	22.56 ± 4.10		0.324 †
RA Area, cm^2	17.70 ± 4.90	15.78 ± 3.32		0.068 ‡
RVd basal, cm	3.59 ± 0.70	3.40 ± 0.49		0.280 ‡
RVd mid, cm	2.42 ± 0.47	2.39 ± 0.43		0.848 †
RVd long, cm	6.24 ± 0.82	6.37 ± 0.70		0.496 ‡
FAC, %	43.32 ± 7.14	45.39 ± 6.38		0.253 ‡

TR, tricuspid regurgitation; PPM, permanent pacemaker; AV, atrioventricular; LVEF, left ventricular ejection fraction; LVIDd, left ventricular internal dimension in diastole; LAVI, left atrial volume index; TAPSE, tricuspid annular plane systolic excursion; LVIDs, left ventricular internal dimension in systole; RA, right atrium; RVd basal, right ventricular basal diameter at end-diastole; RVd mid, right ventricular mid diameter at end-diastole; RVd long, right ventricular longitudinal diameter at end-diastole; FAC, fractional area change; OR, odds ratio; 95% CI, 95% confidence interval. * Chi-square test. † Mann–Whitney test. ‡ Unpaired t-test.

Most pacemaker leads had an inferior position (63.75%) in the RAO view and a septal position (77.5%) in the LAO view. A mid position in the RAO view and septal position in the LAO view were risk factors for worsening TR. A mid-septal position was associated with the highest risk of worsening TR (Table 2). Lead impingement was found in 26.25% of subjects. A fluoroscopic mid position in the RAO view increased the risk of lead impingement ($p < 0.001$). A septal position in the LAO view increased the risk of lead impingement, but this was not statistically significant. Lead impingement was most prevalent in the mid-septal position in the combined RAO–LAO view (Table 3). Further analysis showed that lead impingement was associated with a high risk of significant TR ($p < 0.001$) (Table 4).

Table 2. Association between the pacemaker lead position and significant tricuspid regurgitation ($n = 80$).

Fluoroscopy	Worsening TR ($n = 23$)	Not Worsening TR ($n = 57$)	OR (95% CI)	p-Value
RAO, n (%)				
Mid	14 (60.9)	15 (26.3)	4.36 (1.56–12.13)	**0.04**
Inferior	9 (39.1)	42 (73.7)		
LAO, n (%)				
Septal	21 (91.3)	41 (71.9)	4.10 (0.86–19.52)	0.06
Lateral	2 (8.7)	16 (28.1)		
RAO–LAO, n (%)				
Mid-lateral	0	6 (10.5)		**0.001**
Mid-septal	14 (60.9)	9 (15.8)		
Inferior-lateral	2 (8.7)	10 (17.5)		
Inferior-septal	7 (30.4)	32 (56.1)		
RAO–LAO, n (%)				
Mid-septal	14 (60.9)	9 (15.8)	8.30 (2.76–24.90)	**<0.001**
Others	9 (39.1)	48 (84.2)		

TR, tricuspid regurgitation; RAO, right anterior oblique; LAO, left anterior oblique; OR, odds ratio; 95% CI, 95% confidence interval. Bold values indicate significant results.

Table 3. Association between the pacemaker lead position and lead impingement ($n = 80$).

Fluoroscopy	Impinging ($n = 21$)	Non-Impinging ($n = 59$)	OR (95% CI)	p-Value
RAO, n (%)				
Mid	16 (76.2)	13 (22.0)	11.32 (3.49–36.77)	<0.001
Inferior	5 (23.8)	46 (78.0)		
LAO, n (%)				
Septal	19 (90.5)	43 (72.9)	3.54 (0.74–16.92)	0.097
Lateral	2 (9.5)	16 (27.1)		
RAO-LAO, n (%)				
Mid-Septal	16 (76.2)	7 (11.9)	23.77 (6.63–85.25)	<0.001
Other	5 (23.8)	52 (88.1)		

RAO, right anterior oblique; LAO, left anterior oblique; OR, odds ratio; 95% CI, 95% confidence interval.

Table 4. Association between lead impingement and significant tricuspid regurgitation prevalence ($n = 80$) ($p < 0.001$).

| Lead Impingement | Tricuspid Regurgitation | | OR (95% CI) |
	Worsening ($n = 23$)	Not Worsening ($n = 57$)	
Impinging, n (%)	18 (78.3)	3 (5.3)	64.8 (14.06–298.52)
Non-impinging, n (%)	5 (21.7)	54 (94.7)	

OR, odds ratio; 95% CI, 95% confidence interval.

Based on univariate analysis, there were several variables that fulfilled the requirements for multivariate analysis namely age, sex, hypertension, atrial fibrillation, presence of heart failure, implant duration, mid fluoroscopy position on RAO view, septal fluoroscopy position on LAO, and mid-septal fluoroscopy position in the combined RAO–LAO view. The logistic regression analysis was performed using the backward stepwise elimination method to obtain a final model that had statistical significance. The multivariate analysis showed that a fluoroscopic mid-septal location was a significant predictor of worsening TR ($p = 0.001$; odds ratio [OR], 8.352; 95% confidence interval [CI], 2.514–27.746) In the final model, hypertension and atrial fibrillation were also included as clinical risk factors that were analyzed, of which hypertension was considered a significant risk factor (Table 5).

Table 5. Multivariate analysis.

	Characteristic	β	SE	OR$_{adj}$ (95% CI)	p-Value
First Step	PPM lead position				
	Inferior-septal (ref)	-	-	-	
	Mid-septal	2.558	0.735	12.913 (3.056–54.554)	**0.001**
	Sex	0.638	0.749	1.892 (0.436–8.212)	**0.038**
	Age (years)	−0.006	0.028	0.994 (9.942–1.049)	0.831
	Duration of implantation (months)	0.011	0.008	1.011 (0.005–1.027)	0.175
	Hypertension	1.871	0.903	6.493 (1.106–38.125)	**0.038**
	Atrial fibrillation	1.513	0.762	4.541 (1.021–20.207)	**0.047**
	Coronary heart disease	−1.415	0.850	0.243 (0.046–1.285)	0.096
	Heart failure	0.474	0.668	1.607 (0.434–5.951)	0.478
	Constant	−0.942			
Final Step	Hypertension	1.878	0.858	6.543 (1.218–35.140)	**0.029**
	Atrial fibrillation	1.105	0.640	3.019 (0.862–10.575)	0.084
	Mid-septal position	2.123	0.613	8.352 (2.514–27.746)	**0.001**
	Constant	−3.563			

β, logistic regression coefficient; SE, standard error; OR$_{adj}$, adjusted odds ratio; CI, confidence interval; ref, reference; PPM, permanent pacemaker.

4. Discussion

4.1. Risk Factors for Significant TR

Our study reported a 28.75% progression to significant TR; although this may be considered high, it is within the range of the previously reported incidences of 18.3%, 24.2%, and 39% [11–13]. In our cohort, there were no differences in RA and RV dimensions, TAPSE, and also RV fractional area change (FAC) between those with and without worsening of TR.

The clinical factors associated with worsening TR that were evaluated in our study were age, sex, history of coronary heart disease, hypertension, atrial fibrillation, presence of heart failure, and duration of implantation. The patients with significant TR had a higher mean age, consistent with a previously reported finding that an age between 72 and 75 years was a risk factor for TR [12].

Our study showed a higher prevalence of significant TR for women, but the difference was not statistically significant. Riesenhuber et al. [14] reported an increase in the prevalence of significant TR for women, but this difference might have been caused by differing sample sizes. However, female sex could still be considered a risk factor for TR after PPM implantation.

A history of coronary heart disease was not associated with significant TR. A similar result was reported by another study that found a lower prevalence of significant TR for patients with coronary heart disease; however, this finding was not statistically significant [15].

Hypertension was a predictor of significant TR, and we found a statistically significant association in our study ($p = 0.026$). The mechanism of this in our subjects is unclear since all patients with pulmonary hypertension were excluded. Chronic hypertension could increase left ventricle load resulting in hypertensive cardiac disease, which, if progressive, can develop to left heart failure. Further backflow from the left ventricle to the left atrium may result in diastolic dysfunction, mitral regurgitation, or decreased left atrial compliance. Increased pulmonary arterial hypertension will worsen pulmonary vessel remodeling and can increase the right ventricle load, possibly leading to right ventricle dilatation. At this stage, the risk of TR increases [16,17].

Atrial fibrillation may result in TR in the long term because of right atrial dilatation. Enlargement of the right atrium is followed by annular dilatation [18]. Previous studies showed that TR in the elderly with chronic atrial fibrillation was secondary to right atrial enlargement, right ventricle dysfunction, and tricuspid annulus dilatation, regardless of pulmonary hypertension [19,20]. Although statistically not significant, atrial fibrillation was found in almost 35% of the cohort with worsening TR, compared to only 20% in the cohort without worsening TR. There were no differences in the atrial dimensions (RA area, LA dimension, and LAVI) in both groups.

Our study showed that several lead positions, as identified by fluoroscopy, were risk factors for lead impingement. It is also known that TR is associated with reduced survival rates. Because impingement disturbs tricuspid valve motion and results in significant TR, this finding may predispose patients to right heart failure. With the expanding use and indications of cardiac implantable electronic devices such as pacemakers in bradyarrhythmias, it is important to recognize the remodeling and enlargement of the right heart chambers, which induces further annular dilatation and creating a never-ending cycle of right heart dilatation and worsening TR. A study by Vaturi et al. noted that active right ventricular pacing may increase the severity of TR; the median pacing rate was 100% in the current population [21]. In the present study, right ventricular dyssynchrony as measured by the percentage of right ventricular pacing was not associated with significant TR.

4.2. Association between the Pacemaker Lead Position and Worsening TR

Some mechanisms postulated include perforation, laceration, lead entanglement, or fibrous adherence, thus impairing valve mobility and coaptation [8,11,22–24]. Lead impingement on valve leaflets can also result in mechanical disruption of the valve closure. The pacemaker lead position was evaluated in the RAO view with a 30° angulation and in the LAO view with a 55° angulation using fluoroscopy. Our study showed that certain lead positions significantly increased the prevalence of worsening TR ($p < 0.001$). The highest prevalence of worsening TR was observed in the mid-septal position, and the most prevalent position of leads in all patients was inferior-septal. In the mid-lateral position, we did not observe any significant TR.

A previous study by Poorzand et al. concluded that defining lead positions with fluoroscopy could not predict increased TR severity ($p > 0.05$). In this study, they only used a single antero-posterior view for fluoroscopy without further angulation [25]. In contrast, our study showed that lead positions defined by fluoroscopy using certain angulations could predict significant TR. A mid-septal position increased significant TR; hence, our findings suggest that mid-septal positions should be avoided when placing leads.

4.3. Association between the Pacemaker Lead Position and Lead Impingement Status

There was a significant association between the lead position defined by fluoroscopy and lead impingement as identified by echocardiography. The mid position in the RAO view was a risk factor for lead impingement, as was the septal position in the LAO view. The most prevalent lead impingement was found in the mid-septal position. A study by Addetia et al. showed that the presence of a device lead interfering with normal tricuspid valve leaflet motion was the most significant factor associated with the development of TR after device placement, thus supporting our findings on the impact of lead impingement on significant TR [26].

To reduce the risk of PMTR, it should be ensured that the non-mid-septal position provides enough slack for the pacemaker lead during implantation, thus allowing the lead to move inferiorly. This could be performed using the RAO view with 30° of angulation. The posteroseptal commissure should be the goal of lead placement because TR and lead impingement risks are low when the lead is positioned inside the commissure. When the lead has enough slack to move to a more inferior position, the LAO view with 55° of angulation is useful for ensuring that the lead is placed more septally. It is preferable to position the lead in the posteroseptal commissure of the tricuspid valve to avoid the mid-septal position. This position should be easier to achieve than the mid-lateral and inferior-lateral positions. In the future, it would be beneficial to implant the device leads using 3D TTE guidance.

4.4. Study Limitations

One of the limitations of this study is that our center is a tertiary referral care center, in which patients who underwent echocardiography were more likely to develop symptoms after implantation or other forms of valvular or myocardial dysfunction. Echocardiographic measurements were also not performed in an independent echocardiographic laboratory and interobserver differences regarding the assessment of TR severity may have influenced the results. Other limitations of this study were the relatively small sample size and the various timelines of patient evaluation, which needs to be improved in future studies.

5. Conclusions

We confirmed that PMTR remains a significant problem after pacemaker lead implantation. Only hypertension was found to be a clinical risk factor associated with significant TR. Pacemaker lead positions are adequately visualized by fluoroscopy in the RAO and LAO views. Leads in the mid and septal positions were associated with higher risks of worsening TR and lead impingement. Three-dimensional TTE remains an invaluable tool for assessing tricuspid valve function and may be used to guide future intracardiac device lead implantation procedures.

Author Contributions: Conceptualization, Y.Y.; methodology, Y.Y. and A.M.S.; writing—original draft preparation, D.A.H.; formal analysis, S.I., H., M.A., B.S. and D.A.H.; writing—review and editing, S.I., H., M.A. and D.A.H.; supervision, A.M.S., S.B.R., B.S. and Y.Y. All authors have read and agreed to the published version of the manuscript.

Funding: This research received no external funding.

Institutional Review Board Statement: The study was conducted in accordance with the Declaration of Helsinki, and approved by the Medical Research Ethic Committee of Universitas Indonesia Medical School, Jakarta Indonesia (LB.02.01/VII/441/KEP.049/2020 on June 2020).

Informed Consent Statement: Informed consent was obtained from all subjects involved in the study.

Data Availability Statement: The datasets used and/or analyzed during the current study are available from the corresponding author on reasonable request.

Acknowledgments: The authors thank Michael J. Simorangkir and Dorothy S. Christabella for their help throughout this study.

Conflicts of Interest: The authors declare no conflict of interest.

References

1. Chang, J.D.; Manning, W.J.; Ebrille, E.; Zimetbaum, P.J. Tricuspid Valve Dysfunction Following Pacemaker or Cardioverter-Defibrillator Implantation. *J. Am. Coll. Cardiol.* **2017**, *69*, 2331–2341. [CrossRef] [PubMed]
2. Prihadi, E.A.; van der Bijl, P.; Gursoy, E.; Abou, R.; Mara Vollema, E.; Hahn, R.T.; Stone, G.W.; Leon, M.B.; Ajmone Marsan, N.; Delgado, V.; et al. Development of Significant Tricuspid Regurgitation over Time and Prognostic Implications: New Insights into Natural History. *Eur. Heart J.* **2018**, *39*, 3574–3581. [CrossRef] [PubMed]
3. Delling, F.N.; Hassan, Z.K.; Piatkowski, G.; Tsao, C.W.; Rajabali, A.; Markson, L.J.; Zimetbaum, P.J.; Manning, W.J.; Chang, J.D.; Mukamal, K.J. Tricuspid Regurgitation and Mortality in Patients with Transvenous Permanent Pacemaker Leads. *Am. J. Cardiol.* **2016**, *117*, 988–992. [CrossRef] [PubMed]
4. Seo, Y.; Nakajima, H.; Ishizu, T.; Iida, N.; Sato, K.; Yamamoto, M.; Machino-Ohtsuka, T.; Nogami, A.; Ohte, N.; Ieda, M. Comparison of Outcomes in Patients with Heart Failure with Versus without Lead-Induced Tricuspid Regurgitation after Cardiac Implantable Electronic Devices Implantations. *Am. J. Cardiol.* **2020**, *130*, 85–93. [CrossRef] [PubMed]
5. Mediratta, A.; Addetia, K.; Yamat, M.; Moss, J.D.; Nayak, H.M.; Burke, M.C.; Weinert, L.; Maffessanti, F.; Jeevanandam, V.; Mor-Avi, V.; et al. 3D Echocardiographic Location of Implantable Device Leads and Mechanism of Associated Tricuspid Regurgitation. *JACC Cardiovasc. Imaging* **2014**, *7*, 337–347. [CrossRef] [PubMed]
6. Trankle, C.R.; Gertz, Z.M.; Koneru, J.N.; Kasirajan, V.; Nicolato, P.; Bhardwaj, H.L.; Ellenbogen, K.A.; Kalahasty, G. Severe Tricuspid Regurgitation Due to Interactions with Right Ventricular Permanent Pacemaker or Defibrillator Leads. *Pacing Clin. Electrophysiol.* **2018**, *41*, 845–853. [CrossRef]
7. Andre, C.; Piver, E.; Perault, R.; Bisson, A.; Pucheux, J.; Vermes, E.; Pierre, B.; Fauchier, L.; Babuty, D.; Clementy, N. Galectin-3 Predicts Response and Outcomes after Cardiac Resynchronization Therapy. *J. Transl. Med.* **2018**, *16*, 299. [CrossRef]

8. Lin, G.; Nishimura, R.A.; Connolly, H.M.; Dearani, J.A.; Sundt, T.M., III.; Hayes, D.L. Severe Symptomatic Tricuspid Valve Regurgitation Due to Permanent Pacemaker or Implantable Cardioverter-Defibrillator Leads. *J. Am. Coll. Cardiol.* **2005**, *45*, 1672–1675. [CrossRef]
9. Galiè, N.; Humbert, M.; Vachiery, J.-L.; Gibbs, S.; Lang, I.; Torbicki, A.; Simonneau, G.; Peacock, A.; Vonk Noordegraaf, A.; Beghetti, M.; et al. 2015 ESC/ERS Guidelines for the Diagnosis and Treatment of Pulmonary Hypertension. *Eur. Respir. J.* **2015**, *46*, 903–975. [CrossRef] [PubMed]
10. Zoghbi, W.A.; Adams, D.; Bonow, R.O.; Enriquez-Sarano, M.; Foster, E.; Grayburn, P.A.; Hahn, R.T.; Han, Y.; Hung, J.; Lang, R.M.; et al. Recommendations for Noninvasive Evaluation of Native Valvular Regurgitation. *J. Am. Soc. Echocardiogr.* **2017**, *30*, 303–371. [CrossRef]
11. Kim, J.B.; Spevack, D.M.; Tunick, P.A.; Bullinga, J.R.; Kronzon, I.; Chinitz, L.A.; Reynolds, H.R. The Effect of Transvenous Pacemaker and Implantable Cardioverter Defibrillator Lead Placement on Tricuspid Valve Function: An Observational Study. *J. Am. Soc. Echocardiogr.* **2008**, *21*, 284–287. [CrossRef] [PubMed]
12. Klutstein, M.; Balkin, J.; Butnaru, A.; Ilan, M.; Lahad, A.; Rosenmann, D. Tricuspid Incompetence Following Permanent Pacemaker Implantation. *Pacing Clin. Electrophysiol.* **2009**, *32*, S135–S137. [CrossRef] [PubMed]
13. Seo, Y.; Ishizu, T.; Nakajima, H.; Sekiguchi, Y.; Watanabe, S.; Aonuma, K. Clinical Utility of 3-Dimensional Echocardiography in the Evaluation of Tricuspid Regurgitation Caused by Pacemaker Leads. *Circ. J.* **2008**, *72*, 1465–1470. [CrossRef] [PubMed]
14. Riesenhuber, M.; Spannbauer, A.; Gwechenberger, M.; Pezawas, T.; Schukro, C.; Stix, G.; Schneider, M.; Goliasch, G.; Anvari, A.; Wrba, T.; et al. Pacemaker Lead-Associated Tricuspid Regurgitation in Patients with or without Pre-Existing Right Ventricular Dilatation. *Clin. Res. Cardiol.* **2021**, *110*, 884–894. [CrossRef]
15. Seo, J.; Kim, D.-Y.; Cho, I.; Hong, G.-R.; Ha, J.-W.; Shim, C.Y. Prevalence, Predictors, and Prognosis of Tricuspid Regurgitation Following Permanent Pacemaker Implantation. *PLoS ONE* **2020**, *15*, e0235230. [CrossRef]
16. Prihadi, E.A. Tricuspid Valve Regurgitation: No Longer the "Forgotten Valve". *E-J. Cardiol. Pract.* **2018**, *16*, 21–30.
17. Sysol, J.R.; Machado, R.F. Classification and Pathophysiology of Pulmonary Hypertension. *Contin. Cardiol. Educ.* **2018**, *4*, 2–12. [CrossRef]
18. Nemoto, N.; Lesser, J.R.; Pedersen, W.R.; Sorajja, P.; Spinner, E.; Garberich, R.F.; Vock, D.M.; Schwartz, R.S. Pathogenic Structural Heart Changes in Early Tricuspid Regurgitation. *J. Thorac. Cardiovasc. Surg.* **2015**, *150*, 323–330. [CrossRef]
19. Utsunomiya, H.; Itabashi, Y.; Mihara, H.; Berdejo, J.; Kobayashi, S.; Siegel, R.J.; Shiota, T. Functional Tricuspid Regurgitation Caused by Chronic Atrial Fibrillation. *Circ. Cardiovasc. Imaging* **2017**, *10*, e004897. [CrossRef]
20. Najib, M.Q.; Vinales, K.L.; Vittala, S.S.; Challa, S.; Lee, H.R.; Chaliki, H.P. Predictors for the Development of Severe Tricuspid Regurgitation with Anatomically Normal Valve in Patients with Atrial Fibrillation. *Echocardiography* **2012**, *29*, 140–146. [CrossRef]
21. Vaturi, M.; Kusniec, J.; Shapira, Y.; Nevzorov, R.; Yedidya, I.; Weisenberg, D.; Monakier, D.; Strasberg, B.; Sagie, A. Right Ventricular Pacing Increases Tricuspid Regurgitation Grade Regardless of the Mechanical Interference to the Valve by the Electrode. *Eur. J. Echocardiogr.* **2010**, *11*, 550–553. [CrossRef] [PubMed]
22. Paniagua, D.; Aldrich, H.R.; Lieberman, E.H.; Lamas, G.A.; Agatston, A.S. Increased Prevalence of Significant Tricuspid Regurgitation in Patients with Transvenous Pacemakers Leads. *Am. J. Cardiol.* **1998**, *82*, 1130–1132. [CrossRef]
23. Al-Mohaissen, M.A.; Chan, K.L. Prevalence and Mechanism of Tricuspid Regurgitation Following Implantation of Endocardial Leads for Pacemaker or Cardioverter-Defibrillator. *J. Am. Soc. Echocardiogr.* **2012**, *25*, 245–252. [CrossRef]
24. Lee, R.C.; Friedman, S.E.; Kono, A.T.; Greenberg, M.L.; Palac, R.T. Tricuspid Regurgitation Following Implantation of Endocardial Leads: Incidence and Predictors. *Pacing Clin. Electrophysiol.* **2015**, *38*, 1267–1274. [CrossRef] [PubMed]
25. Poorzand, H.; Tayyebi, M.; Hosseini, S.; Heidari, A.; Keihanian, F.; Jarahi, L.; Hamedanchi, A. Effect of Right Ventricular Lead Placement on Tricuspid Valve: Added Value of Post-Procedural Fluoroscopy to Three Dimensional Echocardiography in a Prospective Cohort Study. *Authorea Prepr.* **2020**. [CrossRef]
26. Addetia, K.; Maffessanti, F.; Mediratta, A.; Yamat, M.; Weinert, L.; Moss, J.D.; Nayak, H.M.; Burke, M.C.; Patel, A.R.; Kruse, E.; et al. Impact of Implantable Transvenous Device Lead Location on Severity of Tricuspid Regurgitation. *J. Am. Soc. Echocardiogr.* **2014**, *27*, 1164–1175. [CrossRef] [PubMed]

Disclaimer/Publisher's Note: The statements, opinions and data contained in all publications are solely those of the individual author(s) and contributor(s) and not of MDPI and/or the editor(s). MDPI and/or the editor(s) disclaim responsibility for any injury to people or property resulting from any ideas, methods, instructions or products referred to in the content.

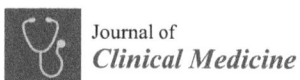 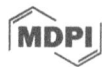

Article

Electroanatomical Mapping System-Guided vs. Intracardiac Echocardiography-Guided Slow Pathway Ablation: A Randomized, Single-Center Trial

Botond Bocz, Dorottya Debreceni, Kristof-Ferenc Janosi, Marton Turcsan, Tamas Simor and Peter Kupo *

Heart Institute, Medical School, University of Pecs, Ifjusag Utja 13, H-7624 Pécs, Hungary; boczbotond@gmail.com (B.B.); debreceni.d@gmail.com (D.D.); janosikristof32@gmail.com (K.-F.J.); marcittm@gmail.com (M.T.); tsimor@hotmail.com (T.S.)
* Correspondence: peter.kupo@gmail.com; Tel.: +36-72-536001; Fax: +36-72-536-387

Abstract: Radiofrequency (RF) catheter ablation is an effective treatment option for targeting the slow pathway (SP) in atrioventricular nodal reentry tachycardia (AVNRT). Previous data suggested that using intracardiac echocardiography (ICE) guidance could improve procedural outcomes when compared to using fluoroscopy alone. In this prospective study, we aimed to compare the effectiveness of an electroanatomical mapping system (EAMS)-guided approach with an ICE-guided approach for SP ablation. Eighty patients undergoing SP ablation for AVNRT were randomly assigned to either the ICE-guided or EAMS-guided group. If the procedural endpoint was not achieved after 8 RF applications; patients were allowed to crossover to the ICE-guided group. The ICE-guided approach reduced the total procedure time (61.0 (56.0; 66.8) min vs. 71.5 (61.0; 80.8) min, $p < 0.01$). However, the total fluoroscopy time was shorter (0 (0–0) s vs. 83.5 (58.5–133.25) s, $p < 0.001$) and the radiation dose was lower (0 (0–0) mGy vs. 3.3 (2.0–4.7) mGy, $p < 0.001$) with EAMS-guidance. The ICE-guided group had a lower number of RF applications (4 (3–5) vs. 5 (3.0–7.8), $p = 0.03$) and total ablation time (98.5 (66.8–186) s vs. 136.5 (100.5–215.8) s, $p = 0.02$). Nine out of 40 patients (22.5%) in the EAMS-guided group crossed over to the ICE-guided group, and they were successfully treated with similar RF applications in terms of number, time, and energy compared to the ICE-guided group. There were no recurrences during the follow-up period. In conclusion, the utilization of ICE guidance during SP ablation has demonstrated notable reductions in procedural time and RF delivery when compared to procedures guided by EAMS. In challenging cases, an early switch to ICE-guided ablation may be the optimal choice for achieving successful treatment.

Keywords: electroanatomical mapping systems; intracardiac echocardiography; slow pathway ablation; AVNRT

1. Introduction

Atrioventricular nodal reentrant tachycardia (AVNRT) is the predominant type of paroxysmal supraventricular tachycardia (SVT), which is characterized by reentry circuitry in the atrioventricular (AV) node region [1]. Although the precise circuitry underlying AVNRT remains unclear, existing evidence indicates that the inferior nodal extensions likely act as the substrate for conduction through the slow pathway (SP) [1].

The catheter ablation procedure targeting the slow pathway (SP) is widely recognized as a primary therapeutic approach for the management of AVNRT. It has consistently exhibited favorable outcomes with high success rates in both the short-term and long-term follow-up periods. However, in certain cases, the ablation of the SP can present challenges due to anatomical variations [2,3].

In SP ablation procedures, the placement of the ablation catheter is guided by anatomical considerations, and intracardiac electrograms are used to ensure accuracy [4,5]. Traditionally, fluoroscopy-guided catheter positioning was employed during the ablations.

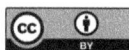

However, the advent of electroanatomical mapping systems (EAMS) over the last decades has demonstrated their superior efficacy compared to fluoroscopy-guided techniques, particularly in reducing fluoroscopy exposure during SP ablations [6–8].

Intracardiac echocardiography (ICE) is an exceptional imaging technique that provides real-time visualization of intracardiac structures, as well as the position and stability of the ablation catheter [9,10].

Previous research has shown that utilization of ICE guidance during SP ablation procedures results in a noteworthy reduction in mapping and ablation time, radiation exposure, and radiofrequency (RF) energy delivery. These findings highlight the advantages of using ICE guidance over fluoroscopy-only procedures [11].

Despite the utility of ICE and EAMS in SP ablation procedures for AVNRT, no scientific data currently exist comparing the efficacy of these two techniques. Consequently, our aim was to perform a study comparing the procedural outcomes of ICE-guided and EAMS-guided SP ablation in patients undergoing this procedure (Figure 1).

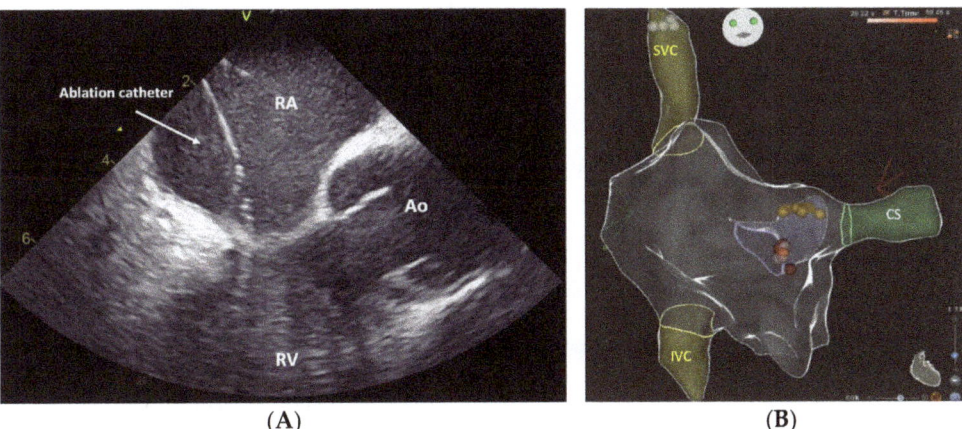

Figure 1. Panel (**A**): Intracardiac echocardiography (ICE) enables the direct observation of the ablation catheter within the region of the slow pathway. Panel (**B**): Three-dimensional electroanatomical map for slow pathway ablation. Abbreviations: Ao, aortic root; CS, coronary sinus; IVC, inferior vena cava; RA, right atrium; RV, right ventricle; and SVC, superior vena cava.

2. Methods

2.1. Study Population

In our single-center trial (registration number: NCT05907863), we recruited 80 patients consecutively who were scheduled to undergo an electrophysiology (EP) study and SP RF ablation for AVNRT. These patients were randomly assigned to two groups: ICE-guided or EAMS-guided ablation groups. The procedures were performed by an experienced electrophysiologist who possessed expertise and proficiency in utilizing both ICE and EAMS for SP ablations. Patients who were referred for a second procedure had other arrhythmias in addition to AVNRT or were under 18 years old were excluded from the study. The study was conducted in accordance with the Declaration of Helsinki and was approved by the regional ethics committee. All patients provided written informed consent to participate in the study.

2.2. Study Protocol

To prepare for the EP study, antiarrhythmic drugs were discontinued at least five half-lives before the procedure, and were under conscious sedation using midazolam ± fentanyl while fasting.

2.3. ICE-Guided Ablation Group

In patients randomized to the ICE-guided ablation group, catheter placement was initially performed using fluoroscopy guidance, after local anesthesia. A decapolar steerable catheter (ViaCath 10, Biotronik, Berlin, Germany) was placed in the coronary sinus (CS), a quadripolar electrode (Triguy, APTMedical, Shenzen, China) catheter was positioned in the right ventricular apex and an ablation catheter (Biotronik AlCath LT G FullCircle, Biotronik, Germany) was inserted to record the His bundle electrogram. During the study, twelve-lead electrocardiogram (ECG) and intracardiac electrograms were acquired and stored using a digital recording system. The recordings were filtered using a band pass filter with a frequency range of 30 to 500 Hz. In order to test AV nodal conduction and induce AVNRT, electrical stimulation techniques were employed.

A stepwise approach was followed during the study where the S2 coupling interval, which refers to the time interval between two consecutive electrical stimulations, was systematically decreased after each drive-train stimulation. The goal was to provoke specific outcomes, such as inducing tachycardia, observing AV conduction block, or reaching the refractory period of the atria. The process involved a gradual reduction in the S2 coupling interval until one of these predefined endpoints was achieved. In cases where tachycardia was not successfully induced during the initial stimulation protocol, an isoprenaline infusion was administered. The infusion aimed to raise the heart rate by a minimum of 20%. Following the infusion, the same stimulation protocol was repeated, encompassing both the infusion and subsequent washout phases.

The diagnosis of AVNRT was made using established electrophysiologic criteria and pacing maneuvers. The methods involved assessing the A-(H)-V response after ventricular overdrive pacing and measuring the SA-VA interval. A SA-VA interval greater than 85 ms was considered indicative of AVNRT. Additionally, the corrected postpacing interval minus the tachycardia cycle length was calculated, and a value greater than 110 ms supported the diagnosis of AVNRT [12,13].

After confirmation of the diagnosis of AVNRT through the diagnostic EP study, the quadripolar electrode catheter was removed and exchanged with an 8F ICE catheter (AcuNaV™ 90 cm, Siemens Medical Solutions, Mountain View, CA, USA) to facilitate both mapping and SP ablation. To enable clear visualization of the anatomical landmarks, the ICE was positioned within the low right atrium, specifically at the 6 o'clock position (Supplementary Videos S1–S4). Subsequently, the catheter was gently rotated in a clockwise direction towards the septum of the heart. This rotational movement ensured optimal imaging and identification of the relevant anatomical structures during the procedure. The distance between the ablation catheter and the compact AV node was assessed by measuring the distance from the aortic valve. The aortic valve serves as a reference point that indicates the recording site of a proximal His potential. This measurement technique helped determine the proximity of the ablation catheter to the compact AV node, ensuring accurate placement during the procedure. In cases of ineffective ablation, the catheter was moved closer to the aortic valve, but a distance of at least 0.5 cm was always maintained, and RF application was attempted again. RF energy was administered beginning just below the CS. The power output for RF energy delivery was set at 30 Watts, and a preset temperature of 55 °C was used as a target during the ablation process. Effective applications were continued for 30 to 60 s and considered successful when junctional rhythm appeared. In the event of catheter displacement, sudden impedance rise, prolongation of PR interval, anterograde AV block, or retrograde ventriculoatrial (VA) block, the delivery of RF energy was promptly ceased. These parameters were monitored closely during the procedure, and any of these signs or events indicated the need to halt the RF application to ensure patient safety and minimize potential complications.

2.4. EAMS-Guided Ablation Group

In the EAMS group, the operator's intention was to carry out fluoroscopy-free procedures. An ablation catheter (NAVISTAR, Biosense Webster, CA, USA) was inserted into the heart to create an anatomical map by CARTO3 EAMS of the right atrium after local anesthesia, and the location of the His bundle was tagged. Decapolar and quadripolar diagnostic catheters were subsequently positioned in their appropriate locations as previously described. Notably, this was achieved without the use of fluoroscopy. Once the diagnosis of AVNRT was established, the mapping of the SP started using a NAVISTAR catheter guided by EAMS. The mapping was performed by assessing the atrial-to-ventricular electrogram amplitude ratio, with a desired range of 1:3 to 1:5. If the ablation endpoint was not reached after 8 radiofrequency (RF) applications, patients in the EMAS-guided ablation group were allowed to crossover to an ICE-guided procedure.

The ablation procedure was deemed successful if, following a 20-min waiting period, the arrhythmia failed to be induced and there were no instances of more than one echo beat observed, both in the presence and absence of isoprenaline.

The duration of the procedure was calculated by measuring the time elapsed from the initial femoral puncture, which marked the beginning of the intervention, until the withdrawal of the catheters, which indicated the conclusion of the procedure. The mapping plus ablation time was determined by measuring the duration starting from the initiation of the slow pathway (SP) mapping until the completion of the final attempted ablation. The fluoroscopy system automatically recorded the duration of fluoroscopy time, radiation dose, and dose-area product (DAP). The ablation data, including the total number of RF applications, cumulative RF energy delivered in watt-seconds (Ws), and the overall ablation time in seconds, were calculated and stored by the electrophysiology (EP) recording system (CardioLab, GE Healthcare, Chicago, IL, USA). The follow-up time was defined as the duration from the procedure to the last telemedicine ambulatory visit. All patients included in the study completed the full 1-year follow-up period. No instances of patient loss occurred during the study.

2.5. Statistical Analysis

The distribution pattern of the data was evaluated using Kolmogorov–Smirnov tests, which assessed the conformity of the data to a specific probability distribution. All statistical tests conducted were two-tailed, and a significance level of $p < 0.05$ was considered statistically significant. Continuous data were presented as mean ± standard deviation (SD) or median with interquartile range (IQR), depending on the appropriateness of the data distribution. Categorical variables were expressed as absolute numbers and percentages. For comparisons between groups, the chi-square test was used for categorical variables, while the T-test and Mann–Whitney U test were employed for continuous variables, depending on the nature of the data. All statistical analyses were performed using SPSS 24 software, developed by SPSS Inc. located in Chicago, IL, USA.

3. Results

We enrolled 80 patients in our study, with 40 patients assigned to the EAMS-guided group and 40 patients to the ICE-guided SP ablation group. There were no significant differences in baseline characteristics, including sex (female: 70.0% vs. 67.5%, $p = 0.81$) and age (49.6 ± 14.9 vs. 53.0 ± 13.4 years, $p = 0.15$), between the groups (Table 1). All 80 cases achieved the procedural endpoint, resulting in a 100% acute success rate. However, the ICE-guided group had significantly shorter procedure time (61.0 (56.0; 66.8) min vs. 71.5 (61.0; 80.8) min, $p < 0.01$), puncture to mapping time (32.5 ± 8.5 min vs. 40.3 ± 10.2 min, $p < 0.01$), and mapping plus ablation time (3 (2; 10.25) min vs. 6.5 (3; 20.5) min, $p = 0.04$).

In contrast, the EAMS-guided group had significantly lower total fluoroscopy time (0 (0–0) s vs. 83.5 (58.5–133.25) s, $p < 0.001$) and total fluoroscopy exposure (0 (0–0) mGy vs. 3.3 (2.0–4.7) mGy, $p < 0.001$) due to the absence of fluoroscopy use during the procedures (no fluoroscopy use was required). Furthermore, after inserting the ICE catheter in the ICE-guided group, fluoroscopy was not necessary. The total ablation time (98.5 (66.8–186) s vs. 136.5 (100.5–215.8) s, $p = 0.02$) and the number of RF applications (4 (3–5) vs. 5 (3.0–7.8), $p = 0.03$) were also lower in the ICE-guided group, although no significant difference was found in the sum of delivered RF energy (3052 (2027–5070) Ws vs. 3572 (2591–6210) Ws, $p = 0.16$) between the two groups.

Table 1. Procedural parameters in the study population.

	ICE-Guided	EAMS-Guided	p-Value
Puncture to mapping time (min)	32.5 ± 8.5	40.3 ± 10.2	<0.001
Mapping plus ablation time (min)	3 (2; 10.25)	6.5 (3; 20.5)	0.04
Total procedure time (min)	61 (56.0; 66.8)	71.5 (61.0; 80.8)	0.004
Fluoroscopy time (s)	83.5 (58.5; 133.25)	0 (0; 0)	<0.001
Fluoroscopy dose (mGy)	3.3 (2.0; 4.7)	0 (0; 0)	<0.001
Radiation exposure (Gycm2)	0.41 (0.27; 0.72)	0 (0; 0)	<0.001
Number of RF applications	4 (3; 5)	5 (3; 7.8)	0.03
Total ablation time (s)	98.5 (66.8; 186.0)	136.5 (100.5; 215.8)	0.02
Sum of delivered energy (Ws)	3052 (2027; 5070)	3572 (2591; 6209.5)	0.16
Fluoroscopy time from diagnosis to the end of the procedure (s)	0 (0; 0)	0 (0; 0)	1
Fluoroscopy dose from diagnosis to the end of the procedure (mGy)	0 (0; 0)	0 (0; 0)	1
Radiation exposure from diagnosis to the end of the procedure (Gycm2)	0 (0; 0)	0 (0; 0)	1

RF, Radiofrequency; ICE, Intracardiac echocardiography; EAMS, Electroanatomical mapping system.

In the EAMS-guided group, a total of 9 out of 40 patients (22.5%) were crossed over to the ICE-guided group based on the operator's discretion, as specified in the methods section. This decision was made due to the failure to achieve the ablation endpoint after 8 RF applications: despite a favorable response to the ablation (junctional acceleration) in 5 cases, the original arrhythmia remained inducible. In 3 cases, junctional acceleration could not be achieved. Following the crossover, in 4 cases, a steerable sheath was introduced to enhance the stability of the ablation catheter. After the crossover, all patients were treated successfully with similar RF applications in terms of number, time, and cumulative energy compared to the ICE-guided group, as shown in Table 2. No complications occurred during the study, and there were no instances of recurrence during the 12.8 ± 3.2-month follow-up period.

Table 2. Procedural parameters in the crossover group.

	Crossover Group
Fluoroscopy time from CO (min)	0 (0; 0)
Fluoroscopy dose from CO (mGy)	0 (0; 0)
Radiation exposure from CO (Gycm2)	0 (0; 0)
Ablation time from CO (s)	103 (90; 122)
Number of RF applications from CO	4 (3; 6)
Sum of delivered energy from CO (Ws)	2673 (2100; 3368)

CO, Crossover; RF, Radiofrequency.

4. Discussion

In this randomized comparative study evaluating the outcomes of EAMS-guided versus ICE-guided ablation of the SP for AVNRT, our findings indicate that the use of ICE is advantageous in reducing the duration of mapping and ablation procedures, minimizing unnecessary RF energy delivery, and enabling successful treatment of complex cases.

The conventional method for ablation of the SP using fluoroscopy guidance is highly effective but poses significant risks related to radiation exposure for both the operating personnel and the patients. Continuous exposure to radiation can result in increased risks of cataracts, dermatitis, and cancer due to both stochastic and deterministic effects [14–16]. To reduce the above-mentioned risk of fluoroscopy, in recent years different zero/minimal-fluoroscopic (Z/MF) techniques have been developed.

EAMS utilizes specialized software to track the position of catheters within the heart, providing a 3D map of the atrial cavity that can be manipulated for optimal visualization. This technology can provide information regarding the location and depth of the applied lesions, as well as details about components of the conduction system (e.g., His bundle). However, it should be noted that the ability of EAMS to accurately represent anatomic variations is limited [7,17,18].

The implementation of EAMSs in ablation procedures enables the use of a Z/MF strategy, thereby eliminating radiation hazards for both patients and personnel. Multiple studies have previously conducted comparisons between the Z/MF fluoroscopy strategy and the conventional approach in the treatment of AVNRTs [7,19,20]. Studies have shown, that catheter ablation for AVNRT without fluoroscopic guidance is feasible and safe, and does not prolong procedure time. A recent meta-analysis that included 24 studies and 9074 patients compared the efficacy of Z/MF and conventional approaches in treating SVT. The analysis found that the use of EAMS significantly reduced radiation dose, fluoroscopy time, and ablation time. However, EAMS guidance had no significant impact on total procedural time, acute and long-term success rates, or complication rates [21].

In certain situations, the utilization of steerable sheaths may be necessary during SVT ablations. However, this has previously posed a challenge to the application of the Z/MF strategy. The recent development of visualizable steerable sheaths which can be tracked by EAMSs, has improved procedural outcomes by allowing for the implementation of the Z/MF strategy even in cases where steerable sheaths are required [22].

Although EAMSs can effectively decrease both fluoroscopy time and dose, they may not be as useful in identifying anatomical variations since they lack direct visualization of anatomical structures. ICE is an advanced imaging modality that enables the dynamic visualization of intracardiac structures in real time. The ICE-guided method provides a clear and immediate visual representation of the heart, allowing for the detection of potential anatomic variations within the Koch-triangles area. This area is known to vary significantly in terms of both anatomy and electrophysiology between individuals [23,24].

According to a previously published randomized trial, ICE-guided SP ablation has been found to have advantages over the conventional fluoroscopic method. Specifically, the use of ICE guidance resulted in reduced total fluoroscopy time and radiation exposure, as well as a reduction in total ablation time, energy requirements, and the number of necessary ablation applications. Notably, due to the study protocol, a quarter of the patients in the fluoroscopy group switched to the ICE-guided group. Nevertheless, all patients were effectively treated exhibiting comparable numbers of RF applications, durations of the procedure, and cumulative RF energy delivery in comparison to the ICE group [11].

Consistent with these findings, our study has provided evidence that integrating ICE guidance during RF ablation of the SP not only reduces the need for radiation exposure during the procedure but also reduces unnecessary RF energy delivery. This is achieved by offering a clear visualization of both the ablation catheter and the targeted SP region, enabling more precise and targeted ablation without the reliance on fluoroscopy.

The observed decrease in RF energy delivery may potentially influence the occurrence of late conduction disturbances following the procedure [25]. Remarkably, even in challenging procedures initially guided by EAMS but subsequently crossed over ICE guidance, comparable quantities, durations, and cumulative energy of RF applications were necessary when compared to the group guided solely by ICE. The crossover rate to ICE in the EAM-guided cases was observed to be 22.5%. This crossover rate is comparable to the rate found in a previous study that compared fluoroscopy-guided and ICE-guided SP ablations [11]. This implies that using ICE to directly visualize the target area and catheter during SP ablation is just as effective, even in cases of unusual anatomy. Importantly, four individuals successfully completed the procedure using a steerable catheter. This observation suggests that the efficacy of the procedure might be more closely linked to the stability of the catheter rather than the specific guidance method employed, whether it be EAM or ICE.

In our opinion, the decision to employ a steerable sheath can be expedited through the use of ICE, as the visualization offered by ICE distinctly reveals instances of unstable catheter–tissue contact. Such scenarios, if uncorrectable through conventional methods, may necessitate the use of a steerable sheath.

It is noteworthy to emphasize that the utilization of ICE in the context of AVNRT ablation bestows a unique advantage through its ability to enhance the visualization of intracardiac structures, thereby augmenting procedural precision. However, it is imperative to duly recognize that intracardiac signals hold a pivotal role in guiding the accurate positioning of the catheter during the procedure.

The sole potential drawback to using an ICE-guided approach for SP ablation is the increased cost associated with the utilization of the catheter. However, this expense is comparable to or even lower than the cost of using an EAMS, especially when using reprocessed ICE catheters [26,27]. In comparison to an EAMS, ICE may offer the additional benefit of more precise ablation targeting with reduced energy delivery, as well as facilitating treatment of more complex cases.

5. Limitations

The applicability of this study may be limited to the specific center where it was conducted, as it was a single-center study with a limited number of patients. Furthermore, due to the lack of blinding, the results may have been subject to bias. Noteworthy is that the study protocol did not aim to primarily demonstrate the difference in fluoroscopy use between the ICE and EAMS groups, as ICE was used exclusively for mapping and ablation purposes. All procedures were performed by a single operator who had experience and familiarity with the use of ICE for SP ablations. We acknowledge that our center has accumulated substantial expertise in ICE-guided procedures, which might have contributed to the observed outcomes. This expertise may have influenced the outcomes and procedural success rates observed in the study. Therefore, the results may not necessarily reflect the outcomes that would be obtained by operators with varying levels of experience or expertise in ICE-guided procedures. These limitations should be taken into consideration when interpreting the findings of our study.

6. Conclusions

Utilizing ICE guidance for anatomical SP ablation presents notable advantages over EAMS-guided procedures. These benefits include decreased mapping and ablation time, as well as reduced RF energy delivery. When EAMS-guided ablation is unsuccessful despite a reasonable attempt, transitioning to ICE-guided ablation can be a recommended alternative.

Supplementary Materials: The following supporting information can be downloaded at: https://www.mdpi.com/article/10.3390/jcm12175577/s1, Supplementary Video S1: The ablation catheter enters the right atrium via the inferior vena cava. Supplementary Video S2: Mapping with the ablation catheter occurs at the His region, where the septal leaflet of the tricuspid valve and the aortic root are interconnected. Supplementary Video S3: Unstable ablation catheter position when mapping slow pathway. Supplementary Video S4: Achieving a stabilized catheter position with an ablation catheter in the region of the slow pathway.

Author Contributions: B.B., D.D., K.-F.J. and M.T. collected the procedural data. The ablation procedures and statistical analysis were conducted by P.K., D.D., K.-F.J. and B.B. contributed to the arrhythmia diagnosis and assisted during the procedures. The study was designed by P.K. and B.B. was responsible for the main data registry and for the interpretation of the results. B.B. and P.K. wrote and revised the paper. P.K. and T.S. served as scientific advisors. The final approval was given by P.K. All authors have read and agreed to the published version of the manuscript.

Funding: This research received no external funding.

Institutional Review Board Statement: The study was performed in accordance with the Declaration of Helsinki and was evaluated following institutional guidelines.

Informed Consent Statement: Informed consent was obtained from all subjects involved in the study.

Data Availability Statement: The data presented in this study are available on request from the corresponding author. The data are not publicly available due to Hungarian legal regulations.

Conflicts of Interest: The authors declare no conflict of interest.

References

1. Katritsis, D.G.; Camm, A.J. Atrioventricular Nodal Reentrant Tachycardia. *Circulation* **2010**, *122*, 831–840. [CrossRef]
2. Brugada, J.; Katritsis, D.G.; Arbelo, E.; Arribas, F.; Bax, J.J.; Blomstrom-Lundqvist, C.; Calkins, H.; Corrado, D.; Deftereos, S.G.; Diller, G.P.; et al. 2019 ESC Guidelines for Themanagement of Patients with Supraventricular Tachycardia. *Eur. Heart J.* **2020**, *41*, 655–720. [CrossRef]
3. Kaneko, Y.; Tamura, S.; Kobari, T.; Hasegawa, H.; Nakajima, T.; Ishii, H. Atrioventricular Ring Tachycardias: Atypical Fast-Slow Atrioventricular Nodal Reentrant Tachycardia and Atrial Tachycardia Share a Common Arrhythmogenic Substrate—A Unifying Proposal. *Rev. Cardiovasc. Med.* **2022**, *23*, 369. [CrossRef]
4. Jackman, W.M.; Beckman, K.J.; McClelland, J.H.; Wang, X.; Friday, K.J.; Roman, C.A.; Lazzara, R. Treatment of Supraventricular Tachycardia Due to Atrioventricular Nodal Reentry by Radiofrequency Catheter Ablation of Slow-Pathway Conduction. *N. Engl. J. Med.* **1992**, *327*, 313–318. [CrossRef]
5. Wu, D.; Yeh, S.J.; Wang, C.C.; Wen, M.S.; Lin, F.C. A Simple Technique for Selective Radiofrequency Ablation of the Slow Pathway in Atrioventricular Node Reentrant Tachycardia. *J. Am. Coll. Cardiol.* **1993**, *21*, 1612–1621. [CrossRef]
6. De Ponti, R.; Salerno-Uriarte, J.A. Non-Fluoroscopic Mapping Systems for Electrophysiology: The "tool or Toy" Dilemma after 10 Years. *Eur. Heart J.* **2006**, *27*, 1134–1136. [CrossRef]
7. Álvarez, M.; Tercedor, L.; Almansa, I.; Ros, N.; Galdeano, R.S.; Burillo, F.; Santiago, P.; Peñas, R. Safety and Feasibility of Catheter Ablation for Atrioventricular Nodal Re-Entrant Tachycardia without Fluoroscopic Guidance. *Heart Rhythm.* **2009**, *6*, 1714–1720. [CrossRef]
8. Smith, G.; Clark, J.M. Elimination of Fluoroscopy Use in a Pediatric Electrophysiology Laboratory Utilizing Three-Dimensional Mapping. *PACE—Pacing Clin. Electrophysiol.* **2007**, *30*, 510–518. [CrossRef]
9. Tardif, J.C.; Vannan, M.A.; Miller, D.S.; Schwartz, S.L.; Pandian, N.G. Potential Applications of Intracardiac Echocardiography in Interventional Electrophysiology. *Am. Heart J.* **1994**, *127*, 1090–1094. [CrossRef]
10. Kalman, J.M.; Olgin, J.E.; Karch, M.R.; Lesh, M.D. Use of Intracardiac Echocardiography in Interventional Electrophysiology. *PACE—Pacing Clin. Electrophysiol.* **1997**, *20*, 2248–2262. [CrossRef]
11. Kupo, P.; Saghy, L.; Bencsik, G.; Kohari, M.; Makai, A.; Vamos, M.; Benak, A.; Miklos, M.; Raileanu, G.; Schvartz, N.; et al. Randomized Trial of Intracardiac Echocardiography-Guided Slow Pathway Ablation. *J. Interv. Card. Electrophysiol.* **2022**, *63*, 709–714. [CrossRef]
12. Katritsis, D.G.; Josephson, M.E. Differential Diagnosis of Regular, Narrow-QRS Tachycardias. *Heart Rhythm.* **2015**, *12*, 1667–1676. [CrossRef]
13. Kupó, P.; Tutuianu, C.I.; Kaninski, G.; Gingl, Z.; Sághy, L.; Pap, R. Limitations of Ventricular Pacing Maneuvers to Differentiate Orthodromic Reciprocating Tachycardia from Atrioventricular Nodal Reentry Tachycardia. *J. Interv. Card. Electrophysiol.* **2022**, *63*, 323–331. [CrossRef]
14. Roguin, A.; Goldstein, J.; Bar, O.; Goldstein, J.A. Brain and Neck Tumors among Physicians Performing Interventional Procedures. *Am. J. Cardiol.* **2013**, *111*, 1368–1372. [CrossRef]
15. Reeves, R.R.; Ang, L.; Bahadorani, J.; Naghi, J.; Dominguez, A.; Palakodeti, V.; Tsimikas, S.; Patel, M.P.; Mahmud, E. Invasive Cardiologists Are Exposed to Greater Left Sided Cranial Radiation: The BRAIN Study (Brain Radiation Exposure and Attenuation during Invasive Cardiology Procedures). *JACC Cardiovasc. Interv.* **2015**, *8*, 1197–1206. [CrossRef]
16. Monaco, M.G.L.; Carta, A.; Tamhid, T.; Porru, S. Anti-X Apron Wearing and Musculoskeletal Problems among Healthcare Workers: A Systematic Scoping Review. *Int. J. Environ. Res. Public Health* **2020**, *17*, 5877. [CrossRef]
17. Suleiman, M.; Gepstein, L.; Roguin, A.; Beyar, R.; Boulos, M. Catheter Ablation of Cardiac Arrhythmias Guided by Electroanatomic Imaging (CARTO): A Single-Center Experience. *Isr. Med. Assoc. J.* **2007**, *9*, 260.
18. Sommer, P.; Kircher, S.; Rolf, S.; Richter, S.; Doering, M.; Arya, A.; Bollmann, A.; Hindricks, G. Non-Fluoroscopic Catheter Tracking for Fluoroscopy Reduction in Interventional Electrophysiology. *J. Vis. Exp.* **2015**, *2015*, e52606. [CrossRef]
19. Swissa, M.; Birk, E.; Dagan, T.; Naimer, S.A.; Fogelman, M.; Einbinder, T.; Bruckheimer, E.; Fogelman, R. Radiofrequency Catheter Ablation of Atrioventricular Node Reentrant Tachycardia in Children with Limited Fluoroscopy. *Int. J. Cardiol.* **2017**, *236*, 198–202. [CrossRef]

20. Walsh, K.A.; Galvin, J.; Keaney, J.; Keelan, E.; Szeplaki, G. First Experience with Zero-Fluoroscopic Ablation for Supraventricular Tachycardias Using a Novel Impedance and Magnetic-Field-Based Mapping System. *Clin. Res. Cardiol.* **2018**, *107*, 578–585. [CrossRef]
21. Debreceni, D.; Janosi, K.; Vamos, M.; Komocsi, A.; Simor, T.; Kupo, P. Zero and Minimal Fluoroscopic Approaches During Ablation of Supraventricular Tachycardias: A Systematic Review and Meta-Analysis. *Front. Cardiovasc. Med.* **2022**, *9*, 856145. [CrossRef] [PubMed]
22. Janosi, K.; Debreceni, D.; Janosa, B.; Bocz, B.; Simor, T.; Kupo, P. Visualizable vs. Standard, Non-Visualizable Steerable Sheath for Pulmonary Vein Isolation Procedures: Randomized, Single-Centre Trial. *Front. Cardiovasc. Med.* **2022**, *9*, 1033755. [CrossRef]
23. Yamaguchi, T.; Tsuchiya, T.; Nagamoto, Y.; Miyamoto, K.; Sadamatsu, K.; Tanioka, Y.; Kadokami, T.; Murotani, K.; Takahashi, N. Anatomical and Electrophysiological Variations of Koch's Triangle and the Impact on the Slow Pathway Ablation in Patients with Atrioventricular Nodal Reentrant Tachycardia: A Study Using 3D Mapping. *J. Interv. Card. Electrophysiol.* **2013**, *37*, 111–120. [CrossRef]
24. Chu, E.; Fitzpatrick, A.P.; Chin, M.C.; Sudhir, K.; Yock, P.G.; Lesh, M.D. Radiofrequency Catheter Ablation Guided by Intracardiac Echocardiography. *Circulation* **1994**, *89*, 1301–1305. [CrossRef]
25. Kesek, M.; Lindmark, D.; Rashid, A.; Jensen, S.M. Increased Risk of Late Pacemaker Implantation after Ablation for Atrioventricular Nodal Reentry Tachycardia: A 10-Year Follow-up of a Nationwide Cohort. *Heart Rhythm.* **2019**, *16*, 1182–1188. [CrossRef]
26. Winkle, R.A.; Mead, R.H.; Engel, G.; Kong, M.H.; Patrawala, R.A. Physician-Controlled Costs: The Choice of Equipment Used for Atrial Fibrillation Ablation. *J. Interv. Card. Electrophysiol.* **2013**, *36*, 157–165. [CrossRef]
27. Bank, A.J.; Berry, J.M.; Wilson, R.F.; Lester, B.R. Acceptance Criteria for Reprocessed AcuNav® Catheters: Comparison Between Functionality Testing and Clinical Image Assessment. *Ultrasound Med. Biol.* **2009**, *35*, 507–514. [CrossRef]

Disclaimer/Publisher's Note: The statements, opinions and data contained in all publications are solely those of the individual author(s) and contributor(s) and not of MDPI and/or the editor(s). MDPI and/or the editor(s) disclaim responsibility for any injury to people or property resulting from any ideas, methods, instructions or products referred to in the content.

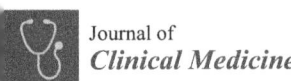

Article

Intracardiac Echocardiography Guidance Improves Procedural Outcomes in Patients Undergoing Cavotricuspidal Isthmus Ablation for Typical Atrial Flutter

Marton Turcsan, Kristof-Ferenc Janosi, Dorottya Debreceni, Daniel Toth, Botond Bocz, Tamas Simor and Peter Kupo *

Heart Institute, Medical School, University of Pecs, Ifjusag utja 13, H-7624 Pecs, Hungary; marcittm@gmail.com (M.T.); janosikristof32@gmail.com (K.-F.J.); debreceni.d@gmail.com (D.D.); dani.toth0319@gmail.com (D.T.); boczbotond@gmail.com (B.B.); tsimor@hotmail.com (T.S.)
* Correspondence: kupo.peter@pte.hu; Tel.: +36-72-536-001; Fax: +36-72-536-387

Abstract: Atrial flutter (AFL) represents a prevalent variant of supraventricular tachycardia, distinguished by a macro-reentrant pathway encompassing the cavotricuspid isthmus (CTI). Radiofrequency (RF) catheter ablation stands as the favored therapeutic modality for managing recurring CTI-dependent AFL. Intracardiac echocardiography (ICE) has been proposed as a method to reduce radiation exposure during CTI ablation. This study aims to comprehensively compare procedural parameters between ICE-guided CTI ablation and fluoroscopy-only procedures. A total of 370 consecutive patients were enrolled in our single-center retrospective study. In 151 patients, procedures were performed using fluoroscopy guidance only, while 219 patients underwent ICE-guided CTI ablation. ICE guidance significantly reduced fluoroscopy time (73 (36; 175) s vs. 900 (566; 1179) s; $p < 0.001$), fluoroscopy dose (2.45 (0.6; 5.1) mGy vs. 40.5 (25.7; 62.9) mGy; $p < 0.001$), and total procedure time (70 (52; 90) min vs. 87.5 (60; 102.5) min; $p < 0.001$). Total ablation time (657 (412; 981) s vs. 910 (616; 1367) s; $p < 0.001$) and the time from the first to last ablation (20 (11; 36) min vs. 40 (25; 55) min; $p < 0.01$) were also significantly shorter in the ICE-guided group. Acute success rate was 100% in both groups, and no major complications occurred in either group. ICE-guided CTI ablation in patients with AFL resulted in shorter procedure times, reduced fluoroscopy exposure, and decreased ablation times, compared to the standard fluoroscopy-only approach.

Keywords: intracardiac echocardiography; cavotricuspidal isthmus; CTI ablation; atrial flutter; ablation

1. Introduction

Atrial flutter (AFL) is a common form of supraventricular tachycardia distinguished by the presence of a macro-reentrant circuit encompassing the cavotricuspidal isthmus (CTI), which denotes a narrow segment of tissue linking the tricuspid valve and the inferior vena cava [1].

For patients experiencing recurrent and symptomatic CTI-dependent AFL, the preferred initial therapeutic approach is radiofrequency (RF) catheter ablation. This procedure aims to establish a bidirectional conduction block across the CTI and exhibits a high degree of success in both short-term and long-term outcomes, with minimal occurrence of complications [2]. Despite the generally favorable efficacy of catheter ablation for CTI, it can be particularly challenging in some cases, frequently attributed to anatomical reasons [3].

Conventionally, electrophysiology procedures have been routinely conducted by employing fluoroscopy guidance, which exposes both patients and medical personnel to potentially hazardous doses of ionizing radiation [4]. In the context of catheter ablation procedures, intracardiac echocardiography (ICE) serves as a unique imaging technique that facilitates the immediate visualization of intracardiac structures in real-time (Figure 1).

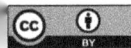

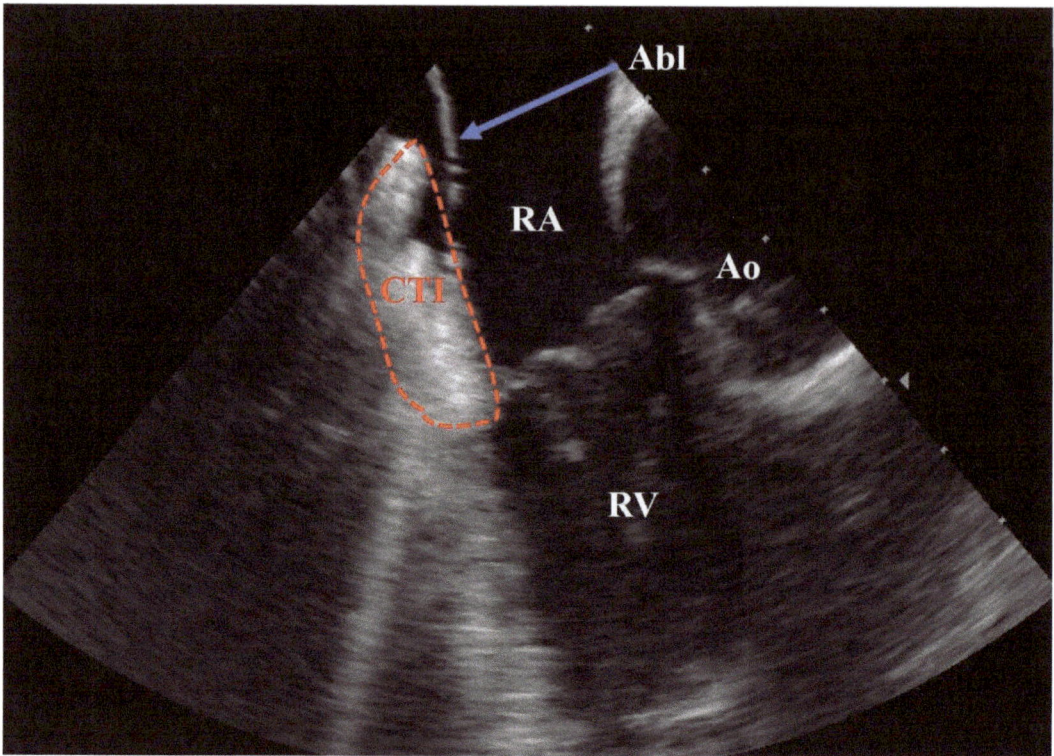

Figure 1. ICE recording during a CTI ablation procedure. Abbreviations: Abl = ablation catheter; CTI = cavotricuspid isthmus; RA = right atrium; RV = right ventricle; Ao = aortic root.

Prior randomized clinical trials demonstrated that the utilization of ICE for CTI ablations significantly decreases radiation exposure in comparison with the fluoroscopy-only procedure. However, the data derived from the studies exhibited inconsistent findings concerning the effects of ICE-guided CTI ablation on procedural time and ablation time [5,6].

Therefore, the objective of our study was to comprehensively compare procedural parameters between the group undergoing CTI ablation guided by ICE and the group guided exclusively by fluoroscopy.

2. Materials and Methods

2.1. Study Population

In our retrospective, single-center study, we enrolled 370 patients who had undergone RF CTI ablation for either ongoing or documented typical AFL at our university hospital from January 2016 to January 2023. Patients included were divided into two groups based on whether ICE had been used during the procedure (ICE group and No ICE group), and the groups were compared on this basis.

We excluded patients referred for a second (redo) procedure, those who had previously undergone atrial fibrillation (AF) ablation or cardiac surgery, and individuals on whom procedures other than CTI ablation had been performed, due to different arrhythmias. We also excluded crossover cases in which ICE was not initially employed at the beginning of the procedure but was subsequently introduced following unsuccessful achievement of the procedural endpoint.

The study protocol adhered to the principles of the Declaration of Helsinki. Consent was obtained in accordance with the ethics research board of our institution. All patients underwent a baseline clinical assessment that encompassed their medical history, electrocardiography (ECG), routine blood tests, and echocardiogram.

2.2. CTI Ablation Procedure

The electrophysiological study and catheter ablation procedures were carried out under conscious sedation using midazolam and fentanyl, with patients in a fasting state and maintained on an uninterrupted anticoagulation regimen. The procedures were conducted by four skilled electrophysiologists who possessed a restricted background in ICE-guided CTI ablation techniques but held considerable expertise in performing fluoroscopy-guided CTI ablations. Subsequent to local anesthesia, following femoral venous access, a decapolar steerable catheter with an interelectrode spacing of 2-5-2 mm (Dynamic Deca, Bard Electrophysiology, Lowell, MA, USA) was positioned within the coronary sinus (CS). Additionally, a 7F irrigated 4 mm tip ablation catheter was inserted into the right atrium (Alcath Black Flux G, Biotronik, Berlin, Germany). The utilization of the 8F ICE catheter (AcuNaV™ 90 cm, Siemens Medical Solutions, Mountain View, CA, USA) was determined by the operators' discretion. The echocardiographic transducer was situated within the inferior right atrium, specifically at the 6 o'clock orientation, with the possibility of lateral adjustment or orientation towards the septum as required. This positioning of the imaging plane facilitated the observation of anatomical reference points within the inferior right atrium, encompassing structures such as the CTI, the CS ostium, the tricuspid valve, the right ventricle, and the Eustachian valve (Supplementary Video S1). In instances where ICE was employed, an extra femoral vein puncture was carried out at the initiation of the procedure. No electroanatomical mapping system was used during the procedures.

In cases of ongoing arrhythmias, entrainment mapping was executed to confirm the cavotricuspidal dependence of the flutters. After discontinuation of the arrhythmia through RF ablation, the procedure was finalized under CS stimulation. For individuals presenting documented typical AFL yet manifesting a normal sinus rhythm during the procedures, ablation was carried out during continuous proximal CS pacing. Twelve-lead electrocardiogram recordings and intracardiac electrograms were acquired and archived utilizing a digital recording system (CardioLab, GE Healthcare, Chicago, IL, USA), incorporating a band-pass filter spanning the frequency range of 30 to 500 Hz.

RF ablation was performed to create a linear lesion along the CTI, employing a point-by-point approach during the ablation process. The ablation was performed in a temperature-controlled manner, maintaining a target temperature of 43 °C. Power delivery was confined to 45 W, while irrigation was maintained at a rate of 15 mL/min. The procedural endpoint included three main components: cessation of the arrhythmia, establishment of the bidirectional isthmus block, and the achievement of a comprehensive line of block. This line was characterized by distinct local double potentials placed at considerable intervals along it, indicating an isoelectric line between two sharp potentials as a result of the CTI ablation.

Major complications were defined as pericardial effusion/tamponade or vascular complications (e.g., major hematomas requiring intervention or prolonged hospitalization, atriovenous fistulas, and pseudoaneurysm).

Acute success was defined as the persistence of a bidirectional conduction block along the CTI following a 20 min observation period. The procedure duration, measured in minutes, spanned from the initiation of the first femoral puncture to the withdrawal of the last venous sheath. Therapy duration (in minutes) was measured from the first to the last RF application. Fluoroscopy time, also measured in minutes, and radiation dose were systematically documented by the fluoroscopy system. The duration of ablation (expressed in seconds) was calculated and stored using the EP recording system.

2.3. Statistical Analysis

The assessment of data distribution characteristics was conducted through the utilization of the Shapiro–Wilk tests. All statistical examinations were carried out with a two-tailed approach, adhering to a significance threshold of $p < 0.05$. Continuous data sets were portrayed as either the mean ± standard deviation or as the median accompanied by the interquartile range, contingent upon the appropriateness of the representation. Conversely, categorical variables were depicted in terms of absolute quantities and corresponding percentages. For the purposes of comparisons, the chi-square test, t test, and Mann–Whitney U test were employed as deemed suitable. The executions of the statistical analyses were facilitated using SPSS 28 software (SPSS, Inc., Chicago, IL, USA).

3. Results

A cumulative cohort of 370 patients were included in the study. Among these, 151 cases underwent exclusively fluoroscopy-guided procedures (designated as the "No ICE group"), while an ICE-guided approach was employed for the remaining 219 patients (referred to as the "ICE group"). The study population comprised 293 male individuals (constituting 79.2% of the total). There were no substantial disparities observed in terms of baseline characteristics between the two groups, with the exception of a lower prevalence of previously diagnosed AF in the No ICE group (68 out of 151 patients (45.6%)), compared to the ICE group (74 out of 219 patients (33.8%), $p = 0.02$). Detailed baseline characteristics of the study population are delineated in Table 1.

Table 1. Demographic and baseline characteristics of the study groups. Abbreviations: EF—ejection fraction; ICE—intracardiac echocardiography; LA—left atrium; TIA—transient ischemic attack.

	No ICE Group (n = 151)	ICE Group (n = 219)	p Value
Age (years)	65.4 ± 10.2	66.5 ± 10.1	0.31
Male (%)	115 (76.2)	178 (81.3)	0.23
Hypertension (%)	113 (74.8)	156 (71.2)	0.33
Diabetes mellitus (%)	48 (32.2)	61 (27.9)	0.37
Reduced EF heart failure (%)	36 (24.2)	52 (23.7)	0.93
Coronary artery disease (%)	49 (32.9)	61 (27.9)	0.30
Chronic kidney disease (%)	20 (13.6)	24 (11)	0.61
Prior stroke/TIA (%)	11 (7.4)	18 (8.3)	0.76
Atrial fibrillation (%)	68 (45.6)	74 (33.8)	0.02
LA diameter (mm)	56.3 ± 6	58 ± 7	0.16

In each instance, a successful bidirectional isthmus block was achieved after a waiting period of 20 min, resulting in a 100% acute success rate. Notably, procedural time displayed a significant decrease within the ICE-guided cohort (No ICE group: 87.5 (60; 102.5) min vs. ICE group: 70 (52; 90) min, $p < 0.001$). The incorporation of ICE guidance led to a substantial reduction in treatment duration (defined as the time between the first and last ablation), evident through a comparison of 40 (25; 55) minutes to 20 (11; 36) minutes ($p < 0.001$). ICE guidance exhibited a substantial association with marked reductions in fluoroscopy time (900 (566; 1179) s vs. 73 (36; 175) s, $p < 0.001$) and decreased exposure to fluoroscopy (40.5 (25.7; 62.9) mGy vs. 2.45 (0.6; 5.1) mGy, $p < 0.001$). Additionally, the total ablation time experienced a decrease in the ICE group (910 (616; 1367) s vs. 657 (412; 981) s, $p < 0.001$). Importantly, the study population did not encounter any major complications. A summary of the results can be found in Table 2.

Table 2. Procedural parameters in the study population. Abbreviation: ICE—intracardiac echocardiography.

	No ICE Group (n = 151)	ICE Group (n = 219)	p Value
Total procedure time (min)	87.5 (60; 102.5)	70 (52; 90)	<0.001
Total ablation time (s)	910 (616; 1367)	657 (412; 981)	<0.001
Treatment duration (min)	40 (25; 55)	20 (11; 36)	<0.001
Total fluoroscopy time (s)	900 (566; 1179)	73 (36; 175)	<0.001
Total fluoroscopy dose (mGy)	40.5 (25.7; 62.9)	2.45 (0.6; 5.1)	<0.001
Acute success rate (%)	100	100	1.0
Major complication (%)	0	0	NA

NA means not applicable.

4. Discussion

In our single-center, retrospective study, we conducted a comparative analysis of procedural data between two groups: ICE-guided vs. fluoroscopy-guided CTI ablations. Our findings did not reveal any statistically significant differences between the groups in terms of major complications and acute success rate. However, the ICE-guided group exhibited several notable advantages over the fluoroscopy-only group, including shorter procedural time, fluoroscopy exposure, total ablation time, and therapy duration.

Catheter ablation plays a significant role in the long-term treatment of AFL by helping to maintain sinus rhythm. The European Society of Cardiology (ESC) guidelines for the management of patients with supraventricular tachycardia, published in 2019, provide recommendations regarding catheter ablation for AFL. In accordance with these guidelines, catheter ablation is recommended for individuals who undergo symptomatic and recurrent episodes of CTI-dependent flutter. Additionally, the ESC guidelines propose that the consideration of CTI ablation after the initial episode of symptomatic typical AFL should be considered [2].

During catheter ablation of the CTI, the primary objective is to create a continuous ablation line along the CTI, leading to the achievement of bidirectional block. Bidirectional block signifies the complete interruption of electrical conduction in both directions across the CTI, effectively eliminating the reentry circuit responsible for typical AFL. Achieving bidirectional block is considered a suitable endpoint for CTI ablation procedures. The existing body of scientific literature consistently demonstrates the high acute and long-term success rates associated with CTI ablation. Notably, multiple studies have substantiated that CTI ablation achieves a long-term success rate exceeding 90% [2,7–9].

The complex anatomical characteristics of the CTI constitute the primary factor contributing to challenges or limitations in achieving a complete and bidirectional conduction block within this region [3,5]. The intricate anatomical features of the CTI encompass several factors, including the elongated isthmus, prominent Eustachian ridges, and the presence of pouches [10,11]. Numerous publications have established a correlation between these anatomical complexities and various procedural factors. Specifically, an association has been identified between these anatomical variations and increased procedure duration, heightened radiation exposure, and an increased number of RF ablations required during CTI ablation for typical AFL [10,12–14].

The utilization of ICE is highly beneficial for the real-time visualization of cardiac anatomical structures during ablation procedures, particularly in patients with complex anatomies [15]. This imaging modality provides valuable assistance in guiding interventions and addressing the challenges posed by intricate anatomical variations. The application of ICE enables healthcare professionals to obtain enhanced visualization of internal cardiac structures, facilitating accurate catheter navigation and precise placement during ablation procedures. Real-time feedback from ICE aids in identifying critical anatomical landmarks and ensuring optimal catheter positioning, thereby improving the efficacy and safety of the intervention [15]. In addition to its guidance capabilities, the incorporation of

ICE has the advantage of reducing the reliance on fluoroscopy, thereby mitigating the need for excessive fluoroscopy exposure during electrophysiological interventions [3].

Previous clinical trials have demonstrated that the incorporation of ICE during CTI ablations yields a substantial reduction in radiation exposure, compared to fluoroscopy-only procedures. In a prospective study involving 102 patients scheduled for CTI ablation conducted by Bencsik et al., the use of ICE was evaluated as a guiding tool during the procedure. The study aimed to assess the impact of ICE on success rates, procedure time, ablation time, radiation exposure, and complications. The results demonstrated that the ICE-guided group ($n = 50$) exhibited a significantly shorter procedure time, fluoroscopy time, and time spent on RF ablation, compared to the fluoroscopy-only group ($n = 52$). Additionally, the ICE-guided group experienced significantly lower radiation exposure and delivered RF energy, compared to the fluoroscopy-only group. Furthermore, seven patients (13%) in the fluoroscopy-only group crossed over to the ICE-guidance group due to prolonged unsuccessful RF ablation, and all of them were successfully treated. The incidence of vascular complications and recurrences were similar between the two groups [5].

Herman et al. conducted a comparative study involving 79 patients undergoing CTI ablation for typical AFL, comparing the use of the ICE-guided approach versus the fluoroscopy-guided approach [6]. Consistent with the findings of Bencsik et al., the authors reported a reduction in fluoroscopy time associated with the utilization of ICE. Interestingly, two patients in the fluoroscopy-only group required crossover to the ICE-guided approach to achieve a bidirectional conduction block. However, it should be noted that the use of ICE resulted in a longer total procedure time, compared to the fluoroscopy-only method. The observed increase in total procedure time in the ICE-guided group, as reported by the authors, can be attributed to the inclusion of an additional vein puncture, compared to the fluoroscopy-only group. This additional puncture contributed to the overall duration of the procedure.

Consistent with prior trials, our retrospective analysis demonstrated a significant reduction in fluoroscopy time associated with the utilization of ICE. Interestingly, contrary to the findings of the study conducted by Herman et al. and in alignment with the results of Bencsik's study, we also observed a decrease in procedure time in the ICE-guided group. These differences in procedure time may be attributed to variations in the definitions of procedure time. In our study and Bencsik's trial, procedure time was defined as the duration from the initiation of the femoral vein puncture to the withdrawal of the last venous sheath. However, in Herman's study, the total procedure time encompassed the duration until successful hemostasis, incorporating the additional vein puncture and time required for achieving proper hemostasis. The use of ICE in CTI ablation procedures requires an additional venous puncture, potentially increasing the risk of vascular complications, particularly when utilizing larger 11F sheaths. However, it is noteworthy that both previous studies and our analysis consistently reported no significant increase in vascular complications within the ICE group. These findings suggest that the use of ICE, despite the supplementary venous puncture, can be safely performed without a notable elevation in adverse vascular events. Moreover, it is important to highlight that current evidence suggests the significant impact of incorporating vascular ultrasound guidance on reducing the incidence of these complications, even in patients receiving uninterrupted oral anticoagulation therapy [16–18]. Based on our exclusion criteria, we excluded patients who underwent crossover to ICE. Crossover to ICE is typically applied when standard, only-fluoroscopy-guided CTI ablation fails. Consequently, some challenging cases from the original fluoroscopy group were excluded. However, only three patients were excluded based on this criterion, so it did not significantly affect our results.

In recent years, the adoption of electroanatomical mapping systems (EAMS) as an alternative visualization modality in electrophysiology procedures has gained increasing popularity. This trend stems from the potential benefits associated with EAMSs, including the ability to decrease procedural time and minimize or completely eliminate radiation exposure. Multiple studies have provided compelling evidence supporting the feasibility and safety of employing a near-zero or zero-fluoroscopy approach utilizing EAMSs during CTI ablations, including their successful application as an extension to pulmonary vein isolation procedures within a single session [19,20]. Furthermore, the introduction of visualizable steerable sheaths has brought about notable progress in reducing radiation exposure during catheter ablation procedures [21].

Nevertheless, EAMSs have certain limitations in directly visualizing intracardiac structures, rendering them less advantageous for catheter ablation procedures in patients with atypical cardiac anatomy. In contrast, ICE emerges as a real-time imaging modality that overcomes this limitation by providing direct visualization of intracardiac structures, aiding in catheter positioning, stability assessment, and monitoring of lesion formation.

The utilization of ICE in cardiac arrhythmia ablation procedures has demonstrated significant benefits. Studies have consistently reported a substantial reduction in fluoroscopy time, fluoroscopy dose, and overall procedure duration when ICE is incorporated, compared to procedures performed without ICE guidance [22,23]. This highlights the added value of ICE in improving procedural efficiency, reducing radiation exposure, and optimizing outcomes in catheter ablation procedures. Moreover, a recent study has provided evidence demonstrating the feasibility of performing zero-fluoroscopy CTI ablation procedures using only ICE, without the need for EAMS [24]. Larger multicenter trials can evaluate the role of ICE in zero-fluoroscopy CTI ablations, with and without EAMS guidance.

The primary limitation of employing an ICE-guided approach for CTI ablation is the associated incremental cost. However, when compared to the additional expenses involved in utilizing EAMSs, the cost of ICE implementation is found to be comparable or potentially even lower [25], especially if the utilization of reprocessed ICE catheters is permitted [26].

5. Limitations

Some limitations need to be acknowledged. Firstly, the study design is retrospective, which means that the data are being collected and analyzed after the events have occurred. This introduces the potential for selection bias, incomplete data, and difficulties in controlling for confounding variables that might influence the outcomes. Secondly, the study was conducted at a single center, which might limit the generalizability of the findings. Furthermore, the operators' varying experience in using ICE may have had an impact on the results. Patient populations and procedural practices can vary significantly between different medical centers, which could impact the external validity of the study's results. Thirdly, although there were no differences in major complications between the groups, due to the lack of data, minor complications (e.g., hematomas not requiring any intervention) could not be compared. Finally, the study primarily focuses on procedural parameters and does not provide information about long-term clinical outcomes.

6. Conclusions

The utilization of ICE shortened procedure time, reduced fluoroscopy exposure, and decreased ablation time in patients who underwent CTI ablation for typical AFL, compared to the standard fluoroscopy-only approach.

Supplementary Materials: The following supporting information can be downloaded at: https://www.mdpi.com/article/10.3390/jcm12196277/s1, Video S1.

Author Contributions: M.T., D.T., B.B. and K.-F.J. collected the procedural data. The statistical analysis was performed by P.K. The study was designed by M.T. and P.K. M.T., D.D. and D.T. were responsible for the main data registry and for the interpretation of the results. P.K. wrote and revised the paper. P.K. and T.S. served as scientific advisors. The final approval was performed by P.K. All authors have read and agreed to the published version of the manuscript.

Funding: This research received no external funding.

Institutional Review Board Statement: The study was performed in accordance with the Declaration of Helsinki and was evaluated following institutional guidelines.

Informed Consent Statement: Informed consent was obtained from all subjects involved in the study.

Data Availability Statement: The data presented in this study are available upon request from the corresponding author. The data are not publicly available due to Hungarian legal regulations.

Conflicts of Interest: The authors declare no conflict of interest.

References

1. Granada, J.; Uribe, W.; Chyou, P.-H.; Maassen, K.; Vierkant, R.; Smith, P.N.; Hayes, J.; Eaker, E.; Vidaillet, H. Incidence and predictors of atrial flutter in the general population. *J. Am. Coll. Cardiol.* **2000**, *36*, 2242–2246. [CrossRef] [PubMed]
2. Brugada, J.; Katritsis, D.G.; Arbelo, E.; Arribas, F.; Bax, J.J.; Blomström-Lundqvist, C.; Calkins, H.; Corrado, D.; Deftereos, S.G.; Diller, G.-P.; et al. 2019 ESC Guidelines for themanagement of patients with supraventricular tachycardia. *Eur. Heart J.* **2020**, *41*, 655–720. [CrossRef] [PubMed]
3. Bencsik, G. Novel Strategies in the Ablation of Typical Atrial Flutter: Role of Intracardiac Echocardiography. *Curr. Cardiol. Rev.* **2014**, *11*, 127–133. [CrossRef] [PubMed]
4. National Research Council. *Health Risks from Exposure to Low Levels of Ionizing Radiation: BEIR VII Phase 2*; The National Academies Press: Washington, DC, USA, 2006. [CrossRef]
5. Bencsik, G.; Pap, R.; Makai, A.; Klausz, G.; Chadaide, S.; Traykov, V.; Forster, T.; Sághy, L. Randomized trial of intracardiac echocardiography during cavotricuspid isthmus ablation. *J. Cardiovasc. Electrophysiol.* **2012**, *23*, 996–1000. [CrossRef]
6. Herman, D.; Osmancik, P.; Zdarska, J.; Cardiocenter, R.P.; Cardiocenter, P. Routine Use of Intracardiac Echocardiography for Atrial Flutter Ablation is Associated with Reduced Fluoroscopy Time, but Not with a Reduction of Radiofrequency Energy Delivery Time Corresponding Author. Available online: www.jafib.com (accessed on 8 March 2022).
7. Lee, K.W.; Yang, Y.; Scheinman, M.M. Atrial flutter: A review of its history, mechanisms, clinical features, and current therapy. *Curr. Probl. Cardiol.* **2005**, *30*, 121–167. [CrossRef]
8. Pérez, F.J.; Schubert, C.M.; Parvez, B.; Pathak, V.; Ellenbogen, K.A.; Wood, M.A. Long-term outcomes after catheter ablation of cavo-tricuspid isthmus díependent atrial flutter: A meta-analysis. *Circ. Arrhythm. Electrophysiol.* **2009**, *2*, 393–401. [CrossRef]
9. Sawhney, N.S.; Feld, G.K. Diagnosis and Management of Typical Atrial Flutter. *Med. Clin. N. Am.* **2008**, *92*, 65–85. [CrossRef]
10. Shimizu, Y.; Yoshitani, K.; Murotani, K.; Kujira, K.; Kurozumi, Y.; Fukuhara, R.; Taniguchi, R.; Toma, M.; Miyamoto, T.; Kita, Y.; et al. The deeper the pouch is, the longer the radiofrequency duration and higher the radiofrequency energy needed—Cavotricuspid isthmus ablation using intracardiac echocardiography. *J. Arrhythm.* **2018**, *34*, 410–417. [CrossRef]
11. Regoli, F.; Faletra, F.F.; Nucifora, G.; Pasotti, E.; Moccetti, T.; Klersy, C.; Auricchio, A. Feasibility and acute efficacy of radiofrequency ablation of cavotricuspid isthmus-dependent atrial flutter guided by real-time 3D TEE. *JACC Cardiovasc. Imaging* **2011**, *4*, 716–726. [CrossRef]
12. Casella, M.; Russo, A.D.; Pelargonio, G.; Del Greco, M.; Zingarini, G.; Piacenti, M.; Di Cori, A.; Casula, V.; Marini, M.; Pizzamiglio, F.; et al. Near zerO fluoroscopic exPosure during catheter ablAtion of supRavenTricular arrhYthmias: The NO-PARTY multicentre randomized trial. *Europace* **2016**, *18*, 1565–1572. [CrossRef]
13. Scaglione, M.; Caponi, D.; Di Donna, P.; Riccardi, R.; Bocchiardo, M.; Azzaro, G.; Leuzzi, S.; Gaita, F. Typical atrial flutter ablation outcome: Correlation with isthmus anatomy using intracardiac echo 3D reconstruction. *Europace* **2004**, *6*, 407–417. [CrossRef] [PubMed]
14. Da Costa, A.; Faure, E.; Thévenin, J.; Messier, M.; Bernard, S.; Abdel, K.; Robin, C.; Romeyer, C.; Isaaz, K.; T, K.; et al. Effect of isthmus anatomy and ablation catheter on radiofrequency catheter ablation of the cavotricuspid isthmus. *Circulation* **2004**, *110*, 1030–1035. [CrossRef] [PubMed]
15. Enriquez, A.; Saenz, L.C.; Rosso, R.; Silvestry, F.E.; Callans, D.; Marchlinski, F.E.; Garcia, F. Use of intracardiac echocardiography in interventional cardiology working with the anatomy rather than fighting it. *Circulation* **2018**, *137*, 2278–2294. [CrossRef] [PubMed]
16. Sobolev, M.; Shiloh, A.L.; Di Biase, L.; Slovut, D.P. Ultrasound-guided cannulation of the femoral vein in electrophysiological procedures: A systematic review and meta-analysis. *Europace* **2017**, *19*, 850–855. [CrossRef] [PubMed]
17. Kupó, P.; Pap, R.; Sághy, L.; Tényi, D.; Bálint, A.; Debreceni, D.; Basu-Ray, I.; Komócsi, A. Ultrasound guidance for femoral venous access in electrophysiology procedures—Systematic review and meta-analysis. *J. Interv. Card. Electrophysiol.* **2020**, *59*, 407–414. [CrossRef] [PubMed]
18. Kupo, P.; Riesz, T.J.; Saghy, L.; Vamos, M.; Bencsik, G.; Makai, A.; Kohari, M.; Benak, A.; Miklos, M.; Pap, R. Ultrasound guidance for femoral venous access in patients undergoing pulmonary vein isolation: A quasi-randomized study. *J. Cardiovasc. Electrophysiol.* **2023**, *34*, 1177–1182. [CrossRef]
19. Debreceni, D.; Janosi, K.; Vamos, M.; Komocsi, A.; Simor, T.; Kupo, P. Zero and Minimal Fluoroscopic Approaches During Ablation of Supraventricular Tachycardias: A Systematic Review and Meta-Analysis. *Front. Cardiovasc. Med.* **2022**, *9*, 856145. [CrossRef]

20. Debreceni, D.; Janosi, K.; Bocz, B.; Turcsan, M.; Lukacs, R.; Simor, T.; Antolič, B.; Vamos, M.; Komocsi, A.; Kupo, P. Zero fluoroscopy catheter ablation for atrial fibrillation: A systematic review and meta-analysis. *Front. Cardiovasc. Med.* **2023**, *10*, 1178783. [CrossRef]
21. Janosi, K.; Debreceni, D.; Janosa, B.; Bocz, B.; Simor, T.; Kupo, P. Visualizable vs. standard, non-visualizable steerable sheath for pulmonary vein isolation procedures: Randomized, single-centre trial. *Front. Cardiovasc. Med.* **2022**, *9*, 1033755. [CrossRef]
22. Goya, M.; Frame, D.; Gache, L.; Ichishima, Y.; Tayar, D.O.; Goldstein, L.; Lee, S.H.Y. The use of intracardiac echocardiography catheters in endocardial ablation of cardiac arrhythmia: Meta-analysis of efficiency, effectiveness, and safety outcomes. *J. Cardiovasc. Electrophysiol.* **2020**, *31*, 664–673. [CrossRef]
23. Kupo, P.; Saghy, L.; Bencsik, G.; Kohari, M.; Makai, A.; Vamos, M.; Benak, A.; Miklos, M.; Raileanu, G.; Schvartz, N.; et al. Randomized trial of intracardiac echocardiography-guided slow pathway ablation. *J. Interv. Card. Electrophysiol.* **2022**, *63*, 709–714. [CrossRef] [PubMed]
24. Luani, B.; Ismail, A.; Kaese, S.; Pankraz, K.; Schmeisser, A.; Wiemer, M.; Braun-Dullaeus, R.C.; Genz, C. Zero-fluoroscopy ablation of the cavotricuspid isthmus guided by intracardiac echocardiography in patients with typical atrial flutter. *Eur. Heart J.* **2022**, *43*, ehac544.441. [CrossRef]
25. Winkle, R.A.; Mead, R.H.; Engel, G.; Kong, M.H.; Patrawala, R.A. Physician-controlled costs: The choice of equipment used for atrial fibrillation ablation. *J. Interv. Card. Electrophysiol.* **2013**, *36*, 157–165. [CrossRef] [PubMed]
26. Bank, A.J.; Berry, J.M.; Wilson, R.F.; Lester, B.R. Acceptance Criteria for Reprocessed AcuNav® Catheters: Comparison Between Functionality Testing and Clinical Image Assessment. *Ultrasound Med. Biol.* **2009**, *35*, 507–514. [CrossRef] [PubMed]

Disclaimer/Publisher's Note: The statements, opinions and data contained in all publications are solely those of the individual author(s) and contributor(s) and not of MDPI and/or the editor(s). MDPI and/or the editor(s) disclaim responsibility for any injury to people or property resulting from any ideas, methods, instructions or products referred to in the content.

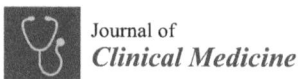 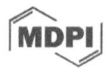

Article

Long-Term Follow-Up of Empirical Slow Pathway Ablation in Pediatric and Adult Patients with Suspected AV Nodal Reentrant Tachycardia

Marta Telishevska *, Sarah Lengauer, Tilko Reents, Verena Kantenwein, Miruna Popa, Fabian Bahlke, Florian Englert, Nico Erhard, Isabel Deisenhofer and Gabriele Hessling

Department of Electrophysiology, German Heart Center Munich, Technical University of Munich, Lazarettstr. 36, 80636 Munich, Germany; lengauer@dhm.mhn.de (S.L.); reents@dhm.mhn.de (T.R.); kantenwein@dhm.mhn.de (V.K.); popa@dhm.mhn.de (M.P.); bahlke@dhm.mhn.de (F.B.); englert@dhm.mhn.de (F.E.); erhard@dhm.mhn.de (N.E.); deisenhofer@dhm.mhn.de (I.D.); hessling@dhm.mhn.de (G.H.)
* Correspondence: martat77@gmail.com; Tel.: +49-(0)89-1218-2020; Fax: +49-(0)89-1218-4593

Abstract: Background: The aim of this study was to assess long-term efficacy and safety of empirical slow pathway (ESP) ablation in pediatric and adult patients with a special interest in patients without dual AV nodal physiology (DAVNP). Methods: A retrospective single-center review of patients who underwent ESP ablation between December 2014 and September 2022 was performed. Follow-up included telephone communication, letter questionnaire and outpatient presentation. Recurrence was based on typical symptoms. Results: 115 patients aged 6–81 years (median age 36.3 years, 59.1% female; 26 pts < 18 years) were included. A typical history was present in all patients (100%), an ECG documentation of narrow complex tachycardia in 97 patients (84%). Patients were divided into three groups: Group 1 without DAVNP ($n = 23$), Group 2 with AH jump ($n = 30$) and Group 3 with AH jump and at least one AV nodal echo beat ($n = 62$). No permanent AV block was observed. During a median follow-up of 23.6 ± 22.7 months, symptom recurrence occurred in 7/115 patients (6.1%) with no significant difference between the groups ($p = 0.73$, log-rank test). Symptom recurrence occurred significantly more often in patients without (5/18 patients; 27%) as compared to patients with ECG documentation (2/97 patients; 2.1%; $p = 0.025$). No correlation between age and success rate was found ($p > 0.1$). Conclusions: ESP ablation is effective and safe in patients with non-inducible AVNRT. Overall, recurrence of symptoms during long-term follow-up is low, even if no DAVNP is present. Tachycardia documentation before the EP study leads to a significantly lower recurrence rate following ESP ablation.

Keywords: atrioventricular nodal reentry tachycardia; dual atrioventricular nodal physiology; empirical slow pathway ablation; recurrence

Citation: Telishevska, M.; Lengauer, S.; Reents, T.; Kantenwein, V.; Popa, M.; Bahlke, F.; Englert, F.; Erhard, N.; Deisenhofer, I.; Hessling, G. Long-Term Follow-Up of Empirical Slow Pathway Ablation in Pediatric and Adult Patients with Suspected AV Nodal Reentrant Tachycardia. *J. Clin. Med.* **2023**, *12*, 6532. https://doi.org/10.3390/jcm12206532

Academic Editor: Ibrahim Marai

Received: 23 August 2023
Revised: 4 October 2023
Accepted: 11 October 2023
Published: 15 October 2023

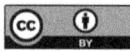

Copyright: © 2023 by the authors. Licensee MDPI, Basel, Switzerland. This article is an open access article distributed under the terms and conditions of the Creative Commons Attribution (CC BY) license (https://creativecommons.org/licenses/by/4.0/).

1. Introduction

Atrioventricular nodal reentry tachycardia (AVNRT) is the most common paroxysmal supraventricular tachycardia (SVT) in adolescents and adults. Catheter ablation is the treatment of choice for symptomatic AVNRT patients. However, the endpoint of the procedure is still not unequivocally established [1]. Catheter ablation for SVT in general, and AVNRT in particular, is the current treatment of choice for symptomatic patients because it substantially improves quality of life [2]. However, in some patients with typical symptoms, no SVT is inducible during the EP study and the final diagnosis of the tachycardia mechanism remains undetermined. In these patients, the ACC/AHA/ESC Guidelines [3] suggest an empirical slow pathway (ESP) ablation under the precondition of (1) existence of a Holter or surface electrocardiographic (ECG) documentation of a tachycardia compatible with AVNRT and (2) documentation of dual atrioventricular nodal pathway physiology (DAVNP) in the form of an AV nodal echo beat and/or an AH jump during programmed atrial stimulation during the EP study.

Studies in adults and some smaller studies in pediatric patients have reported on the long-term outcome of ESP modification under these preconditions [4–10]. Data are lacking about ESP modification in patients with suspected AVNRT without DAVNP during the EP study.

The main threshold to perform ESP ablation in suspected AVNRT is due to the low but not zero risk of ablation-related complete AV block. The clinical relevance of this dilemma is highlighted by a recent survey [7]. In the absence of a characteristic ECG documentation, 44% of the interviewed electrophysiologists stated that it would require a minimum of two echo beats as a threshold to perform ESP, while 19% did not even consider two echo beats as a sufficient indication for slow pathway modification [7]. In another study investigating procedural success and clinical long-term outcome after ESP ablation performed with a minimum of two AV nodal echo beats, the threshold to ablate was lower when a characteristic ECG documentation was present [4].

The aim of this study was to evaluate the long-term outcome after ESP ablation in a large cohort of pediatric and adult patients with suspected, but non-inducible, AVNRT with and without DAVNP in the EP study.

2. Methods

2.1. Study Design

This study was a retrospective analysis of 115 consecutive patients (26 patients < 18 years) who underwent ESP ablation at our institution from December 2014 to September 2022. Baseline characteristics are shown in Table 1. Patients with accessory pathways or with inducible AVNRT during the EP study or during RF delivery at the slow pathway region were excluded.

Table 1. Baseline Characteristics.

Variable	All (n = 115)	Group 1 n = 23 (20%)	Group 2 n = 30 (26%)	Group 3 n = 62 (54%)
Age [yrs], mean ± SD	36.3 ± 18.9	36.8 ± 19.9	34.1 ± 20.9	37.2 ± 17.7
Gender [% female]	68 (59.1)	12 (52.1)	16 (53.3)	40 (64.5)
Patients < 18 yrs (%)	26 (22.6)	4 (17.3)	9 (30)	13 (20.9)
ECG Documentation n (%)	97 (84.3)	16 (69.5)	25 (83.3)	56 (93.3)
Previous EP study without ablation	6 (5.2)	0	2 (6.6)	4 (6.4)
General anesthesia n (%)	3 (2.6)	2 (8.7)	0	1 (1.6)
Conscious sedation n (%)	108 (93.9)	21 (91.3)	27 (90.0)	60 (96.8)
Retrograde conduction n (%)	109 (94.8)	17 (73.9)	18 (60.0)	56 (90.3)
APERP [msec], mean ± SD	332 ± 62	330 ± 52	338 ± 70	334 ± 65
APERP msec after abl, mean ± SD	356 ± 83	357 ± 76	358 ± 93	351 ± 75
3D System n (%):	114 (99.1)			
NaVx	99 (86.1)	20 (86.9)	26 (86.7)	53 (85.4)
Carto 3	15 (13.0)	3 (13.0)	4 (13.3)	8 (12.9)
Atrial fibrillation n (%):	7 (46.6)	3 (13.0)	2 (6.7)	2 (3.2)

All patients fulfilled the following criteria: (1) typical history (typical on—off palpitations) and/or ECG documentation (narrow complex tachycardia with regular cycle length and no discernible P-wave; (2) non-inducibility of AVNRT or other SVT by programmed atrial stimulation with and without pharmacological stimulation; (3) completion of a telephone questionnaire for long-term follow-up.

Patients were divided into 3 groups: Group 1 included patients without AH jump and without AV nodal echo beat(s), Group 2 patients with AH jump without AV nodal echo beat and Group 3 patients with AH jump and 1–2 AV nodal echo beat(s) during the EP study.

The Institutional Ethical Review Board approved the study.

2.1.1. Electrophysiological Study

Electrophysiological studies were performed after written informed consent. All antiarrhythmic drugs had been discontinued at least three half-lives prior to the procedure. The procedure was performed under general anesthesia in pediatric patients < 45 kg (n = 3), analgesia/sedation with propofol and fentanyl (n = 108) or analgesia only with fentanyl (n = 4).

The procedures were performed by four operators with more than 10 years of slow pathway ablation experience utilizing electroanatomical mapping (EAM) systems.

Diagnostic catheters were inserted via transfemoral access and positioned in the coronary sinus, His bundle area, and right ventricle. After placement of catheters, a bolus of 5000 U heparin (pediatric dose 100 U/kg) was administered intravenously. The presence of an accessory pathway was excluded, as described previously [9].

AVNRT induction was attempted using programmed atrial stimulation with 2 basic cycle lengths (600/400 ms or 500/400 ms) followed by 1–3 extrastimuli and additionally by atrial burst stimulation up to a minimum CL of 200 msec. If no tachycardia was induced, orciprenaline (since 2020 isoproterenol) was administered intravenously aiming at a heart rate increase of at least 20% and the stimulation protocol repeated.

Dual atrioventricular nodal physiology (DAVNP) was defined as the presence of any of the following: (1) jump phenomenon as a prolongation of the AH-interval by more than 50 msec after a 10 msec decrease in the coupling interval during programmed extrastimulation; (2) typical slow–fast atrioventricular nodal echo beat; and (3) sustained slow pathway conduction seen during rapid atrial pacing, as described previously [8].

2.1.2. Ablation

A right atrial map was performed using a 3D mapping system in all patients. The expected location of the rightward inferior slow pathway extension was mapped in sinus rhythm at the triangle of Koch, between the posteroseptal tricuspid valve annulus and the ostium of the coronary sinus. Mapping and ablation were performed using a non-irrigated 4-mm tip catheter (Marinr® 7F, Medtronic, Minneapolis, MN, USA; 60°/30W or Navistar® 7F, Biosense, Webster, TX, USA). The catheter was delivered through a standard 8F venous sheath. A long introducer sheath (SR0 ™Fast-Cath™ 8.F, Abbott or SL0 ™Swartz™ 8.5F, Abbott, TX, USA) was used at the discretion of the operator if no stable mapping position was achieved. Non-irrigated RF ablation was targeted at atrioventricular groove sites with a dominant ventricular electrogram and ideally with a "bump-and-spike" atrial electrogram signifying a near-field slow pathway potential. Test radiofrequency applications at target sites were continued for up to 10 s in search junctional rhythm as feedback for effective SP modification. If junctional rhythm at a temperature ≥ 48 °C was achieved, applications were continued for at least 60 s. Applications were terminated if either rapid junctional acceleration (cycle length < 400 ms) or PR interval prolongation was noticed. System impedance measured over the ablation catheter was monitored for evidence of effective tissue heating (10–15 Ω decrease), inadvertent catheter slippage into the coronary sinus or coagulum formation.

2.1.3. Empirical Slow Pathway Ablation

The primary ablation objective was slow junctional rhythm at the target area and a catheter-tip temperature of ≥48 °C. If junctional rhythm with good temperature was noted, RF applications of at least of 60 s were delivered. If no junctional rhythm was observed at various sites, applications were applied corresponding to electrical signals and anatomy. In Group 2 and 3, ablation aimed at eliminating the AH jump and echo beats. However, if lesions were considered effective, as described above, a residual AH jump with one echo beat was tolerated. The atrial stimulation protocol was repeated 20 min following the last ablation.

2.1.4. Post-Ablation Care and Follow-up

In all patients, a transthoracic echocardiogram was performed at the end of the procedure and before discharge. A 12-lead ECG was obtained at the end of the procedure, on the evening of the ablation day and on the day following ablation. A 24-h Holter ECG was obtained before discharge.

In all adult patients, a purse-string suture was applied to venous puncture sites. Venous sheaths were removed directly after purse-string suture, and a groin compression bandage was applied for 6 h. In pediatric patients, venous puncture site compression was performed in the EP lab and a groin compression bandage was implemented for 6 h. All patients received heparin i.v. until removal of bandages. On the day after the ablation procedure, all punctured sites were carefully examined. In the case of abnormalities, an ultrasound evaluation of the femoral vessels was performed.

Follow-up was conducted in our outpatient clinics and by telephone communication with the patient. Clinical outcome was assessed by absence/recurrence of clinical symptoms and/or ECG documentation. Routine ambulatory monitoring was not performed in asymptomatic patients. Time to recurrence was defined as time between procedure and documented tachycardia or recurrence of typical symptoms. Study endpoints were complete elimination of clinical symptoms without documentation of AVNRT recurrence.

3. Statistical Analysis

Mean values were calculated as arithmetic averages and represented as the mean ± SD. Comparisons between groups were made by an unpaired t test or one-way analysis of variance for normally distributed variables. A value of $p < 0.05$ was considered statistically significant. SPSS 23 (SPSS Inc., Chicago, IL, USA) was used for all calculations. For patients with follow-up after initial ablation, freedom from AVNRT recurrence was estimated using the Kaplan–Meier method.

4. Results

4.1. Baseline and Electrophysiological Characteristics

Clinical and electrophysiological characteristics of the patients are shown in Table 1. All patients described typical on—off palpitations and 84.3% of patients (97/115) had ECG documented regular narrow complex tachycardia. Six patients had received a prior EP study without catheter ablation. Median age was 36.33 ± 18.91 years (range 6–81) with 68/115 female patients (59.1%). In four patients, congenital heart disease was present, including cc-TGA with VSD after pulmonary artery banding and tricuspid valve replacement ($n = 1$), bicuspid aortic valve with aortic insufficiency ($n = 1$), aortic stenosis after aortic valve replacement ($n = 1$) and mitral valve disease with mitral insufficiency ($n = 1$). During the EP study, 23/115 pts (20%) showed absence of DAVNP (Group 1), and 30/115 pts (26%) had an AH jump without AV nodal echo beat (Group 2). In 62/115 (54%) patients, DAVNP with AH jump and at least one AV nodal echo beat (7/62 two echo beats) was present. Atrial fibrillation occurred spontaneously or after programmed stimulation in 7/115 (6.6%) patients. No ECG documentation of narrow complex tachycardia was present in 7/23 pts (30.4%) from Group 1, in 5/30 pts (16.7%) from Group 2 and 6/62 pts (9.6%) from Group 3.

4.2. Radiofrequency Ablation

A 3D mapping system was utilized in all patients (n = 115) including the Ensite Velocity/Precision/X™ System (Abbott, TX, USA) in 99 patients (86.1%) or the Carto®3 System (Biosense Webster, TX, USA) in 16 patients (13.9%). In five patients (4.8%), the procedure was performed without fluoroscopy. Junctional rhythm during ablation was noted in 104/115 (90.4%) patients. In Group 1, in 18/23 (78%) patients junctional rhythm was noted during ablation, in Group 2 in 27/30 (90%) patients and in Group 3 in 59/62 (95%) patients ($p > 0.1$). In Group 2, no residual post-ablation AH jump was documented in any patient. In Group 3, a residual AH jump ($n = 5$ pts) or a residual AH jump with one echo beat ($n = 6$ pts) was present.

4.3. Procedure/Ablation Times and Fluoroscopy Time/Dose

Mean procedure time was 81.5 ± 26.3 min (38–170 min) with a mean fluoroscopy time of 3.4 ± 2.8 min (range 0.5–12.5 min) and a mean fluoroscopy dose of 108.7 ± 162.7 cGycm^2 (range 3.78–515.9). Mean RF-time was 4.2 min. Procedure time, fluoroscopy time/dose and RF-time were not significantly different between the groups. Procedural and ablation data are shown in Table 2.

Table 2. Procedural Data.

Variable	All (n = 115)	Group 1 n = 23	Group 2 n = 30	Group 3 n = 62	p Value
Age [yrs], mean ± SD	36.3 ± 18.9	36.8 ± 19.9	34.1 ± 20.9	37.2 ± 17.7	>0.1
Procedure time [min], mean ± SD	81.5 ± 26.3	77.8 ± 28.9	82.9 ± 26.8	82.2 ± 25.4	>0.1
RF-time [min], mean ± SD	4.2 ± 2.8	3.2 ± 1.9	4.3 ± 2.4	4.6 ± 3.2	>0.1
Temperature [grad], mean ± SD	44.5 ± 3.2	44.2 ± 4.3	44.4 ± 2.3	44.6 ± 3.3	>0.1
RF-Energy [watt], mean ± SD	31.8 ± 26.1	26.6 ± 5.9	29.2 ± 5.6	35.3 ± 35.3	>0.1
Fluoro time [min], mean ± SD	3.4 ± 2.8	3.5 ± 2.9	2.7 ± 2.2	3.8 ± 2.9	>0.1
Fluoro dos. [cGycm^2], mean ± SD	108.7 ± 162.7	119.5 ± 167.9	96.5 ± 170.3	110.8 ± 159.3	>0.1

4.4. Safety

Overall mortality was 0%. No intermittent or permanent complete AV block occurred. In Group 3, one major complication was noted in a 69-year-old woman with multiple chronic comorbidities as COPD GOLD IV, postrenal kidney failure, pulmonary embolism and a history of multiple embolic cerebral infarctions. Pericardial effusion was detected 4 h after ablation, probably due to coronary sinus perforation. After successful pericardiocentesis the patient was hemodynamically stable. The pericardial sheath was removed the next day and the patient was discharged 5 days after the ablation in stable condition. In all patients, transthoracic echocardiography at discharge documented normal ventricular function without signs of dyskinesia, thrombi or pericardial effusion. Minor complications were observed in seven patients (6.1%). These included transient first- or second-degree atrioventricular block (n = 4) or right bundle branch block (n = 3), completely resolving by the end of the electrophysiological study. No vascular complications were observed.

4.5. Follow-up

Over a mean observation time of 23.67 ± 22.7 months (3–92 months), seven of 115 patients (6.1%) had recurrence of clinical symptoms. Symptom recurrence occurred in 2/23 patients (8.7%) in Group 1, 2/30 patients (6.7%) in Group 2 and 3/62 patients (4.8%) in Group 3 (Table 3).

Table 3. Symptom recurrence in regard to tachycardia ECG documentation.

Group	No ECG Documentation	Recurrence	Recurrence/No ECG Documentation
1	30.4% (7/23)	8.7% (2/23)	2/2
2	16.7% (5/30)	6.7% (2/30)	2/1
3	9.6% (6/62)	4.8% (3/62)	3/2

Kaplan–Meier analysis shows freedom from AVNRT recurrence without significant difference between the three groups ($p = 0.73$, log-rank test; Figure 1).

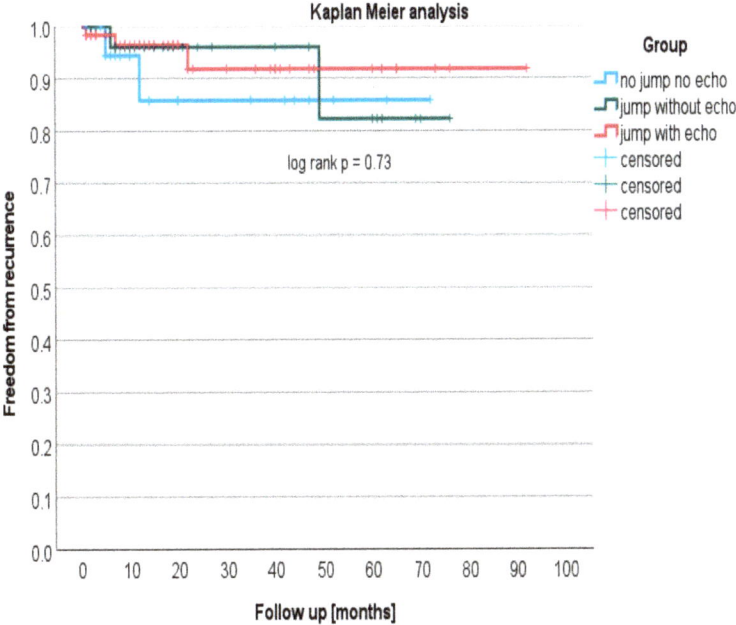

Figure 1. Kaplan–Meier analysis.

No junctional rhythm at ablation had been noted in 4/7 pts (2/2 from Group 1, 2/2 in Group 2 and 0/3 in Group 3) with symptom recurrence. Of the seven patients with symptom recurrence, five patients did not want a second ablation due to rarity of symptoms. Two patients underwent a second SP ablation and interestingly demonstrated AVNRT-induction during the redo procedure (one patient from Group 1 and one patient from Group 2, all without junctional rhythm during the first ablation).

Recurrence rate was significantly higher in patients without prior ECG documentation (5/18 patients; 27%) than in patients with pre-ablation ECG documentation (2/97 patients; 2.1%; $p = 0.025$). In Group 1, 2/2 pts with recurrence from Group 1 were without ECG documentation, 1/2 pts from Group 2, and 2/3 pts from Group 3. This is shown in Table 4.

Table 4. Procedural characteristics and recurrence.

Variable	Recurrence $n = 7$	No Recurrence $n = 108$	p Value
Age [yrs], mean ± SD	33.4 ± 14.2	36.5 ± 19.2	0.60
No ECG Documentation n (%)	5 (71)	13 (12)	0.025
APERP after abl, mean ± SD	360.0 ± 105.0	357.5 ± 82.7	0.95
RF-time [min], mean ± SD	2.2 ± 1.3	4.4 ± 2.8	0.003
Temperature [grad], mean ± SD	46.2 ± 2.5	44.4 ± 3.3	0.14

Pearson's correlation coefficient shows no statistical relationship between younger age and longer RF time ($r = 0.03$) and no correlation between age and success rate of ESP ablation ($p > 0.1$) was found. All 26 pediatric patients and the six patients with prior EP study remained free from symptom recurrence after ESP ablation.

Table 5 shows clinical details of patients reporting symptom recurrence after ESP ablation. No patient required antiarrhythmic drug treatment during follow-up.

Table 5. Clinical details of patients with symptom recurrence after ESP ablation.

	Group	Junctional Rhythm during Abl.	ECG Documentation before Abl.	Frequency of Symptoms before Ablation	ECG Documentation after Abl.	Frequency of Symptoms at FU	Second Ablation for AVNRT	Recurrency at Long-Term FU
Pat. 1	1	No	No	once a month	Yes	once a month	Yes, with AVNRT induction	No
Pat. 2	1	No	No	once a quarter	No	very rare	No	Yes
Pat. 3	2	No	No	twice a week	Yes	once a week	Yes, with AVNRT induction	No
Pat. 4	2	No	Yes	2–3 times/year	No	twice after abl.	No	Yes
Pat. 5	3	Yes	No	1–2 times/year	No	once after abl.	No	Yes
Pat. 6	3	Yes	No	once a month	No	once after abl.	No	Yes
Pat. 7	3	Yes	Yes	once a month	No	twice after abl.	No	Yes

5. Discussion

This large study with 115 patients evaluates empirical slow pathway ablation in symptomatic pediatric and adult patients without inducible AVNRT at the EP study. It is the first study that includes patients with a clinical history consistent with AVNRT but without evidence of dual AV nodal physiology at the EP study. Empirical slow pathway ablation was performed by experienced operators at a high-volume center.

The main finding of the study is that ESP ablation is effective for patients with non-inducible AVNRT and DAVNP, but also for patients without DAVNP in the EP study. The approach is safe and symptom recurrence rate is low, especially in patients with a clinical history consistent with AVNRT and ECG documentation of a regular narrow complex tachycardia before the EP study.

Patients with clinical history consistent with AVNRT but without inducible AVNRT in the EP study still present a problem, as the operator has to decide whether to proceed with ablation. Sluggish antegrade slow-pathway conduction or intermittent suppression of DAVNP due to sedation or other transient factors during the EP study may mask DAVNP. AVNRT inducibility is sometimes complex and requires a perfect balance between slow and fast pathway conduction. However, ESP ablation in non-inducible patients is the only option for a potential cure even in the absence of a clear pre-EP study of short RP tachycardia or DAVNP in an EP study [11].

In a retrospective study by Gerguri et al. [5], 63 patients (19%) with no pre-procedural ECG documentation but DAVNP with a maximum of one echo beat in the EP study were assigned to a "pure" empirical SP group. The other 271 patients (81%) with ECG documentation were assigned to the standard SP group. A higher incidence of other tachycardias and a higher persistence of subjective symptoms were found after pure empirical SP ablation. However, clinical symptoms improved in 60% of patients. The study by He et al. [12] had reported that SP ablation can be performed safely and effectively in non-inducible and suspected AVNRT patients with good long-term results. Also in this study, no tachycardia documentation before ablation was predictive for recurrence. In our study, only 15.6% of patients had no ECG documentation of narrow complex tachycardia. Symptom recurrence was significantly higher in those patients. This be due to the fact that other tachycardia mechanisms (especially focal atrial tachycardia) play a role and ablation did not meet the "real" target.

Our primary ablation objective and endpoint for ablation was sustained slow junctional rhythm with a catheter-tip temperature of ≥ 48 °C. This sustained junctional rhythm as procedural "endpoint" was noted in 90.4% of patients. Shurrab et al. also reported about 90.7% junctional rhythm performing SP ablation [11]. We suggest that slow junctional rhythm could serve as a sufficient endpoint in these cases. Some studies decided DAVNP was a recognized reliable marker of success [13,14], but their results did not show a significant difference to long-term success between junctional rhythm alone versus junctional rhythm plus abolishment of DAVNP as ablation endpoints [14]. Operators do not necessarily need the greater effort and therefore have the greater risk in trying to achieve DAVNP abolishment. The study by Duman et al. showed a non-inducible AVNRT may be accompanied by the absence of some features that represent DAVNP, such as jump, and/or echo beats. The absence of any of these dual AV node features, established before ablation, did not have any effect on outcome [9].

The study by Duman et al. found a procedural success rate of 97.4% and a recurrence rate of 12.6% [9]. In the recent study by O'Leary et al. [15] with 512 pediatric patients with SP ablation for inducible AVNRT, the recurrence rate was 5%. In our study, symptom recurrence after ESP ablation was observed in only 6.1% of patients, which is comparable to the study of Duman. Two patients underwent a second SP ablation and demonstrated AVNRT-induction during a redo of SP ablation; in 5/7 patients, there was a decrease in tachycardia episodes following ESP ablation, and no second ablation was performed [9,16,17].

The main aspects of ESP ablation are safety and efficacy. Although not used in our study, intracardiac echocardiography (ICE) is a technique to avoid or minimize fluoroscopy and increase safety. Potential advantages over 3D EAM are the real-time visualization of true endovascular borders (including duplex-mediated blood flow direction), endocardial structures and diagnostic or ablation catheters, as well as immediate recognition of potential complications (such as pericardial effusion or thrombus formation) [18]. The study by Luani et al. reported that zero-fluoroscopy ICE-guidance shows comparable efficacy and safety when compared to traditional fluoroscopic navigation during cryothermal ablation of the slow pathway in AVNRT patients [18].

The study by Bocz et al. with 80 patients who underwent SP ablation for AVNRT showed no recurrences during follow-up. This study compared ICE guidance and EAM system guidance. Utilizing ICE for anatomical SP ablation showed notable advantages over EAMS-guided procedures [19]. Another study by Kupo et al. demonstrated that ICE-guidance during SP ablation significantly reduces mapping and ablation time, radiation exposure, and RF delivery in comparison to fluoroscopy-only procedures. Moreover, early switching to ICE-guided ablation seems to be an optimal choice in challenging cases [20]. In summary, ICE might present a good alternative to conventional EAM in SP ablation.

In the study by Duman et al. [9] with 79 pediatric patients, the higher prolongation in Wenckebach cycle length and lower mean age were predictors for AVNRT recurrence. In the recent adult study by He et al. [12], a younger age (adolescent age/14–18 years) was related to a higher long-term recurrence rate. We did not find a correlation between age and longer RF time or long-term efficacy of ESP ablation. All pediatric patients in our study showed freedom from symptom recurrence after ESP ablation.

A zero/minimal fluoroscopy approach should be pursued especially in pediatric cases. In our study, in five patients the procedure was performed without fluoroscopy using the Ensite/NavX system. In all the other cases, we aimed for minimal fluoroscopy. In the study by Smith and Clark, zero fluoroscopy was possible in 80% of the procedures, and the use of EAM resulted in a significant decrease in fluoroscopy time [21]. Walsh et al. achieved a complete zero-fluoroscopic approach in 94% (in 47 of 50 pts.) using EAM [22]. The mean fluoroscopy time in our study was higher (3.4 ± 2.8 min) in comparison to the study by Swissa et al. (0.83 ± 1.04 min) using a fluoroscopy-limited approach with a 3D EAM system [23]. The importance of reducing radiation exposure and achieving minimal/zero fluoroscopy procedures is highlighted in the study by Gaita F et. al. [24]. This review summarizes the state of the art of feasibility and safety of the near-to-zero approach for electrophysiological procedures. A meta-analysis by Debreceni et al. reported that a zero/minimal fluoroscopy approach using 3D EAM systems for catheter ablation of SVTs is feasible without compromising acute and long-term success or complication rates [25].

The six patients with previous EP studies with non-inducible AVNRT who underwent ESP ablation also showed freedom from symptom recurrence. In the absence of inducible SVT, some operators may hesitate to perform ESP ablation given the absence of a clear procedural endpoint and the low but not zero risk of complete AV block [26,27]. The difficult decision of whether to perform ESP ablation is a challenge in clinical practice and the perceived need for further evidence to guide this decision is high [7]. Our data suggest that it might be a valid option to extend the indication for ESP ablation beyond the current guidelines to those patients who exhibit DAVNP at the EP study in the absence of tachycardia ECG documentation and to those patients with a clinical history consistent with AVNRT and ECG documentation of tachycardia in the absence of DAVNP. In both cases, it might be advantageous to proceed to ESP ablation to avoid repeat EP studies including possible complications.

6. Conclusions

This study demonstrates that empirical slow pathway ablation in patients with a clinical history consistent with AVNRT with and without tachycardia ECG documentation is a safe procedure with a beneficial outcome for the great majority of the patients. For the first time, it is shown that even patients who do not present with dual-nodal AV physiology in the EP study benefit from the procedure, especially if ECG documentation of narrow complex tachycardia is available. This finding is independent of age; symptomatic children and adolescents without inducible tachycardia may also benefit from empirical slow pathway ablation. Our study might encourage electrophysiologists in high-expertise centers to perform ESP ablation in patients with a clinical history consistent with AVNRT and ECG documentation but without inducible AVNRT even if no DAVNP at the EP study is present.

7. Limitations

The main limitation is the retrospective character of the single-center cohort study with data collection over a longer time period which might include a possible variation in patient management over time. Intravenous sedation as performed at our institution may affect tachycardia inducibility. The use of ICE might further increase safety and efficacy but is currently not available at our center. The recurrence rate was assessed based on clinical parameters only. We cannot completely exclude a placebo effect after ESP ablation.

Author Contributions: Conceptualization, M.T. and S.L.; Methodology, M.T.; Validation, V.K. and M.P.; Formal analysis, T.R., F.B., S.L. and V.K.; Investigation, M.T. and G.H.; Resources, M.P. and T.R.; Data curation, M.T., V.K., S.L., F.B., F.E., N.E. and I.D.; Writing—original draft, M.T.; Writing—review and editing, S.L.; Visualization, S.L. and I.D.; Supervision, G.H.; Project administration, I.D. All authors have read and agreed to the published version of the manuscript.

Funding: This research received no external funding.

Institutional Review Board Statement: Protocol code 2020-348_1-S-NP. Category: clinical study.

Informed Consent Statement: Not applicable.

Data Availability Statement: Not applicable.

Conflicts of Interest: The authors declare no conflict of interest.

References

1. Katritsis, D.G.; Zografos, T.; Siontis, K.C.; Giannopoulos, G.; Muthalaly, R.G.; Liu, Q.; Latchamsetty, R.; Varga, Z.; Deftereos, S.; Swerdlow, C.; et al. Endpoints for successful slow pathway catheter ablation in typical and atypical atrioventricular nodal re-entrant Tachycardia. *JACC Clin. Electrophysiol.* **2019**, *5*, 113–119. [CrossRef]
2. Brugada, J.; Katritsis, D.G.; Arbelo, E.; Arribas, F.; Bax, J.J.; Blomström-Lundqvist, C.; Calkins, H.; Corrado, D.; Deftereos, S.G.; Diller, G.P.; et al. 2019 ESC Guidelines for the management of patients with supraventricular tachycardia. *Eur. Heart J.* **2020**, *41*, 683–685. [CrossRef]

3. Blomström-Lundqvist, C.; Scheinman, M.M.; Aliot, E.M.; Alpert, J.S.; Calkins, H.; Camm, A.J.; Campbell, W.B.; Haines, D.E.; Kuck, K.H.; Lerman, B.B.; et al. ACC/AHA/ESC guidelines for the management of patients with supraventricular arrhythmias–executive summary. *J. Am. Coll. Cardiol.* **2003**, *42*, 1493–1531. [CrossRef]
4. Wegner, F.K.; Silvano, M.; Bögeholz, N.; Leitz, P.R.; Frommeyer, G.; Dechering, D.G.; Zellerhoff, S.; Kochhäuser, S.; Lange, P.S.; Köbe, J.; et al. Slow pathway modification in patients presenting with only two consecutive AV nodal echo. *J. Cardiol.* **2017**, *69*, 471–475. [CrossRef]
5. Gerguri, S.; Jathanna, N.; Lin, T.; Müller, P.; Clasen, L.; Schmidt, J.; Kurt, M.; Shin, D.I.; Blockhaus, C.; Kelm, M.; et al. Clinical impact of "pure" empirical catheter ablation of slow-pathway in patients with non-ECG documented clinical on–of tachycardia. *Eur. J. Med. Res.* **2018**, *23*, 16. [CrossRef]
6. Wegner, F.K.; Bögeholz, N.; Leitz, P.; Frommeyer, G.; Dechering, D.G.; Kochhäuser, S.; Lange, P.S.; Köbe, J.; Wasmer, K.; Mönnig, G.; et al. Occurrence of primarily noninducible atrioventricular nodal reentry tachycardia after radiofrequency delivery in the slow pathway region during empirical slow pathway modulation. *Clin. Cardiol.* **2017**, *40*, 1112–1115. [CrossRef]
7. Laish-Farkash, A.; Shurrab, M.; Singh, S.; Tiong, I.; Verma, A.; Amit, G.; Kiss, A.; Morriello, F.; Birnie, D.; Healey, J.; et al. Approaches to empiric ablation of slow pathway: Results from the Canadian EP web survey. *J. Interv. Card. Electrophysiol.* **2012**, *35*, 183–187. [CrossRef]
8. Pott, C.; Wegner, F.K.; Bögeholz, N.; Frommeyer, G.; Dechering, D.G.; Zellerhoff, S.; Kochhäuser, S.; Milberg, P.; Köbe, J.; Wasmer, K.; et al. Outcome predictors of empirical slow pathway modulation: Clinical and procedural characteristics and long-term follow-up. *Clin. Res. Cardiol.* **2015**, *104*, 946–954. [CrossRef]
9. Duman, D.; Ertuğrul, İ.; Yıldırım Baştuhan, I.; Aykan, H.H.; Karagöz, T. Empiric slow-pathway ablation results for presumed atrioventricular nodal reentrant tachycardia in pediatric patients. *Pacing Clin. Electrophysiol.* **2021**, *44*, 1200–1206. [CrossRef]
10. Emmel, M.; Brockmeier, K.; Sreeram, N. Slow pathway ablation in children with documented reentrant supraventricular tachycardia not inducible during invasive electrophysiologic study. *Z. Kardiol.* **2005**, *94*, 808–812. [CrossRef]
11. Shurrab, M.; Szili-Torok, T.; Akca, F.; Tiong, I.; Kagal, D.; Newman, D.; Lashevsky, I.; Onalan, O.; Crystal, E. Empiric slow pathway ablation in non-inducible supraventricular tachycardia. *Int. J. Cardiol.* **2015**, *179*, 417–420. [CrossRef]
12. He, J.; Liu, Z.; Fang, P.H.; Chen, X.B.; Liu, J.; Tang, M.; Jia, Y.H.; Zhang, S. Long-term efficacy of empirical slow pathway ablation in non-inducible and suspected atrioventricular nodal reentry tachycardia. *Acta Cardiol.* **2016**, *71*, 457–462. [CrossRef]
13. Wagshal, A.B.; Crystal, E.; Katz, A. Patterns of accelerated junctional rhythm during slow pathway catheter ablation for atrioventricular nodal reentrant tachycardia: Temperature dependence, prognostic value, and insights into the nature of the slow pathway. *J. Cardiovasc. Electrophysiol.* **2000**, *11*, 244–254. [CrossRef]
14. Stern, J.D.; Rolnitzky, L.; Goldberg, J.D.; Chinitz, L.A.; Holmes, D.S.; Bernstein, N.E.; Bernstein, S.A.; Khairy, P.; Aizer, A. Meta-analysis to assess the appropriate endpoint for slow pathway ablation of atrioventricular nodal reentrant tachycardia. *Pacing Clin. Electrophysiol.* **2011**, *34*, 269–277. [CrossRef]
15. O'Leary, E.T.; Harris, J.; Gauvreau, K.; Gentry, C.; Dionne, A.; Abrams, D.J.; Alexander, M.E.; Bezzerides, V.J.; DeWitt, E.S.; Triedman, J.K.; et al. Radiofrequency Catheter Ablation for Pediatric Atrioventricular Nodal Reentrant Tachycardia: Impact of Age on Procedural Methods and Durable Success. *J. Am. Heart Assoc.* **2022**, *11*, e022799. [CrossRef]
16. Liuba, I.; Jönsson, A.; Säfström, K.; Walfridsson, H. Gender-related differences in patients with atrioventricular noda lreentry tachycardia. *Am. J. Cardiol.* **2006**, *97*, 384–388. [CrossRef]
17. McCANTA, A.C.; Collins, K.K.; Schaffer, M.S. Incidental dual atrioventricular nodal physiology in children and adolescents: Clinical follow-up and implications. *Pacing Clin. Electrophysiol.* **2010**, *33*, 1528–1532. [CrossRef] [PubMed]
18. Luani, B.; Rauwolf, T.; Genz, C.; Schmeißer, A.; Wiemer, M.; Braun-Dullaeus, R.C. Intracardiac echocardiography versus fluoroscopy for endovascular and endocardial catheter navigation during cryo-ablation of the slow pathway in AVNRT patients. *Cardiovasc. Ultrasound.* **2019**, *17*, 12. [CrossRef]
19. Bocz, B.; Debreceni, D.; Janosi, K.F.; Turcsan, M.; Simor, T.; Kupo, P. Electroanatomical Mapping System-Guided vs. Intracardiac Echocardioraphy-Guided Slow Pathway Ablation: A Randomized, Single-Center Trial. *J. Clin. Med.* **2023**, *12*, 5577. [CrossRef]
20. Kupo, P.; Saghy, L.; Bencsik, G.; Kohari, M.; Makai, A.; Vamos, M.; Benak, A.; Miklos, M.; Raileanu, G.; Schvartz, N.; et al. Randomized trial of intracardiac echocardiography-guided slow pathway ablation. *Interv. Card. Electrophysiol.* **2022**, *63*, 709–714. [CrossRef]
21. Smith, G.; Clark, J.M. Elimination of fluoroscopy use in a pediatric electrophysiology laboratory utilizing three-dimensional mapping. *Pacing Clin. Electrophysiol.* **2007**, *30*, 510–518. [CrossRef] [PubMed]
22. Walsh, K.A.; Galvin, J.; Keaney, J.; Keelan, E.; Szeplaki, G. First experience with zero-fluoroscopic ablation for supraventricular tachycardias using a novel impedance and magnetic-field-based mapping system. *Clin. Res. Cardiol.* **2018**, *107*, 578–585. [CrossRef]
23. Swissa, M.; Birk, E.; Dagan, T.; Naimer, S.A.; Fogelman, M.; Einbinder, T.; Bruckheimer, E.; Fogelman, R. Radiofrequency catheter ablation of atrioventricular node reentrant tachycardia in children with limited fluoroscopy. *Int. J. Cardiol.* **2017**, *236*, 198–202. [CrossRef]
24. Gaita, F.; Guerra, P.G.; Battaglia, A.; Anselmino, M. The dream of near-zero X-rays ablation comes true. *Eur. Heart J.* **2016**, *37*, 2749–2755. [CrossRef]

25. Debreceni, D.; Janosi, K.; Vamos, M.; Komocsi, A.; Simor, T.; Kupo, P. Zero and Minimal Fluoroscopic Approaches During Ablation of Supraventricular Tachycardias: A Systematic Review and Meta-Analysis. *Front. Cardiovasc. Med.* **2022**, *9*, 856145. [CrossRef]
26. Hanninen, M.; Yeung-Lai-Wai, N.; Massel, D.; Gula, L.J.; Skanes, A.C.; Yee, R.; Klein, G.J.; Manlucu, J.; Leong-Sit, P.E.T.E.R. Cryoablation versus RF Ablation for AVNRT: A Meta-Analysis and Systematic Review. *J. Cardiovasc. Electrophysiol.* **2013**, *24*, 1354–1360. [CrossRef] [PubMed]
27. Liao, J.N.; Hu, Y.F.; Wu, T.J.; Fong, A.N.; Lin, W.S.; Lin, Y.J.; Chang, S.L.; Lo, L.W.; Tuan, T.C.; Chang, H.Y.; et al. Permanent Pacemaker Implantation for Late Atrioventricular Block in Patients Receiving Catheter Ablation for Atrioventricular Nodal Reentrant Tachycardia. *J. Cardiol.* **2013**, *111*, 569–573. [CrossRef]

Disclaimer/Publisher's Note: The statements, opinions and data contained in all publications are solely those of the individual author(s) and contributor(s) and not of MDPI and/or the editor(s). MDPI and/or the editor(s) disclaim responsibility for any injury to people or property resulting from any ideas, methods, instructions or products referred to in the content.

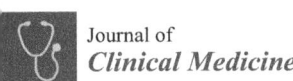

Article

Left Atrial Appendage Occlusion versus Novel Oral Anticoagulation for Stroke Prevention in Atrial Fibrillation—One-Year Survival

Shmuel Tiosano [1,2,†], Ariel Banai [2,3,†], Wesam Mulla [1,4], Ido Goldenberg [1,2], Gabriella Bayshtok [1,2,5], Uri Amit [1,2], Nir Shlomo [1,2], Eyal Nof [1,2], Raphael Rosso [2,3], Michael Glikson [6,7], Victor Guetta [1,2], Israel Barbash [1,2] and Roy Beinart [1,2,*]

1. Leviev Heart Center, Sheba Medical Center, Ramat Gan 52621, Israel; wesam.mulla@sheba.health.gov.il (W.M.)
2. Faculty of Medicine, Tel Aviv University, Ramat Aviv, Tel Aviv 6997801, Israel; arielbanai@gmail.com (A.B.)
3. Department of Cardiology, Tel Aviv Sourasky Medical Center, Tel Aviv 64239, Israel
4. Surgeon General Headquarters, Israel Defense Forces, Ramat Gan 5262000, Israel
5. Arrow Program, Sheba Medical Center, Ramat Gan 5266202, Israel
6. Jesselson Integrated Heart Center, Shaare Zedek Medical Center, Jerusalem 9103102, Israel
7. Faculty of Medicine, Hebrew University of Jerusalem, Jerusalem 9574425, Israel
* Correspondence: roy.beinart@sheba.health.gov.il; Tel.: +972-3-5302608 (ext. 5305330); Fax: +972-3-5305804 (ext. 5356605)
† These authors contributed equally to this work.

Abstract: Aim To compare the 1-year survival rate of patients with atrial fibrillation (AF) following left atrial appendage occluder (LAAO) implantation vs. treatment with novel oral anticoagulants (NOACs). Methods: We have conducted an indirect, retrospective comparison between LAAO and NOAC registries. The LAAO registry is a national prospective cohort of 419 AF patients who underwent percutaneous LAAO between January 2008 and October 2015. The NOACs registry is a multicenter prospective cohort of 3138 AF patients treated with NOACs between November 2015 and August 2018. Baseline patient characteristics were retrospectively collected from coded diagnoses of hospitalization and outpatient clinic notes. Follow-up data was sorted from coded diagnoses and the national civil registry. Subjects were matched according to propensity score. Baseline characteristics were compared using Chi-Square and student's t-test. Survival analysis was performed using Kaplan-Meier survival curves, log-rank test, and multivariable Cox regression, adjusting for possible confounding variables. Results: This study included 114 subjects who underwent LAAO implantation and 342 subjects treated with NOACs. The mean age of participants was 77.9 ± 7.44 and 77.1 ± 11.2 years in the LAAO and NOAC groups, respectively (p = 0.4). The LAAO group had 70 (61%) men compared to 202 (59%) men in the NOAC group (p = 0.74). No significant differences were found in baseline comorbidities, renal function, or CHA_2DS_2-VASc score. One-year mortality was observed in 5 (4%) patients and 32 (9%) patients of the LAAO and NOAC groups, respectively. After adjusting for confounders, LAAO was significantly associated with a lower risk for 1-year mortality (HR 0.38, 95%CI 0.14–0.99). In patients with impaired renal function, this difference was even more prominent (HR 0.21 for creatinine clearance (CrCl) < 60 mL/min). Conclusions: In a pooled analysis of two registries, we found a significantly lower risk for 1-year mortality in patients with AF who were implanted with LAAO than those treated with NOACs. This finding was more prominent in patients with impaired renal function. Future prospective direct studies should further investigate the efficacy and adverse effects of both treatment strategies.

Keywords: left atrial appendage occluder; NOAC; survival; cohort; anticoagulation

Citation: Tiosano, S.; Banai, A.; Mulla, W.; Goldenberg, I.; Bayshtok, G.; Amit, U.; Shlomo, N.; Nof, E.; Rosso, R.; Glikson, M.; et al. Left Atrial Appendage Occlusion versus Novel Oral Anticoagulation for Stroke Prevention in Atrial Fibrillation—One-Year Survival. *J. Clin. Med.* **2023**, *12*, 6693. https://doi.org/10.3390/jcm12206693

Academic Editor: Ibrahim Marai

Received: 6 August 2023
Revised: 6 September 2023
Accepted: 11 September 2023
Published: 23 October 2023

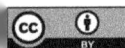

Copyright: © 2023 by the authors. Licensee MDPI, Basel, Switzerland. This article is an open access article distributed under the terms and conditions of the Creative Commons Attribution (CC BY) license (https://creativecommons.org/licenses/by/4.0/).

1. Introduction

Atrial fibrillation (AF), the most common sustained cardiac arrhythmia, affects 3% of the general population and one-fourth of the elderly [1]. It increases the risk of ischemic stroke [2]. Similarly, the prevalence of chronic kidney disease (CKD) increases with age [3], rising to 25% in patients older than 70 [4], and is associated with an increased risk of AF, independent of age [5,6]. Patients with both conditions have a higher risk of ischemic stroke or bleeding [7], making management challenging.

Until a decade ago, warfarin was the preferred drug for preventing ischemic stroke in AF patients [8,9], but it has a narrow therapeutic range, requires frequent monitoring, has numerous drug and food interactions, and poor patient compliance [10]. With the introduction of novel oral anticoagulants (NOACs) for the treatment of non-valvular AF (NVAF) [11–13], the use of warfarin has decreased, except for certain indications such as mechanical heart valve prosthesis or rheumatic mitral valve disease [14]. NOACs have the advantage of not needing monitoring and dose adjustments and fewer interactions with food and drugs.

The optimal anticoagulant for patients with CKD is still a matter of debate, with warfarin being recommended in guidelines [15] but real-world data showing reluctance to prescribe due to bleeding risk and fear of a fatal outcome [16]. NOACs have dose adjustments for CKD patients [17], but randomized trials in severe CKD are lacking. Left atrial appendage occlusion (LAAO) is an alternative invasive treatment with demonstrated benefits in randomized studies and registries [18,19]. The PLAATO trial evaluated the feasibility and safety of LAAO in patients unable to be treated with anticoagulation [20]. The PROTECT AF proved its non-inferiority at one year compared to warfarin [21]. In the follow-up publication, the LAAO showed superiority over warfarin, with reduced total mortality [22]. In the PREVAIL trial, procedural safety was significantly improved compared to PROTECT AF [23]. A Danish study had shown that LAAO might have similar stroke prevention efficacy but a lower risk of major bleeding and mortality [24].

Furthermore, the LAAOS III trial showed promising results in preventing stroke by surgically closing the left atrial appendage during cardiac surgery [25]. In the PRAGUE-17 randomized trial, LAAO was non-inferior to NOACs in preventing major AF-related cardiovascular, neurological and bleeding events, however, without a significant difference in survival [26]. The EHRA/EAPCI currently favor NOACs over LAAO in patients eligible for both treatments due to stronger evidence towards NOACs. Moreover, this position paper questions the PREVAIL study due to the higher rate ratio (1.33, 95% CI 0.78–2.13) of 18-month stroke seen as part of the first co-primary endpoint—a composite of stroke, systemic embolism, and cardiovascular/unexplained death. The recently published SCAI/HRS Expert Consensus Statement on Transcatheter Left Atrial Appendage Closure deems LAAO appropriate when patients are at high thromboembolic risk and not suited for long-term OAC [27]. This study evaluated the efficacy and safety of percutaneous LAAO compared to NOACs in patients with NVAF in an all-comers cohort. Specifically, it evaluated the subpopulation of patients with CKD.

2. Methods

2.1. Patients

This study compared patients who were treated with NOACs and those who were implanted with LAAO. The NOAC group is a pooled sample of 3 different separate multicenter prospective cohorts of consecutive patients treated with a NOAC (either Rivaroxaban $n = 1023$, Apixaban $n = 1164$, and Dabigatran $n = 951$) who entered the study between November 2015 and August 2018. A secure web-based questionnaire produced by the study coordination center at the Israeli Center for Cardiovascular Research was used for data collection. The LAAO database consists of 419 patients with AF who underwent percutaneous LAAO implantation between January 2008 and October 2015. Patients underwent propensity score matching with a 1:3 ratio. The final analysis included 342 patients from the NOAC group and 114 patients in the LAAO group. CrCl for this study was calculated based on the Cockroft-Gault formula.

Devices used for LAA occlusion were either Amplatzer Amulet (Abbott Cardiovascular, Plymouth, MN, USA) or Watchman (Boston Scientific, Marlborough, MA, USA). The decision on which type of device would be installed was based on the operating physicians' preference and clinical characteristics. Usually, patients were discharged with a dual antiplatelet therapy consisting of Aspirin and Clopidogrel for six weeks, followed by a lifelong monotherapy with Aspirin. Most patients who underwent LAAO occlusion had contraindications for anticoagulant treatment.

2.2. Endpoints

The primary endpoint evaluated all-cause mortality at one year. Subgroup analysis of the primary endpoint for different baseline covariates, including renal function, was then executed. Secondary endpoints included ischemic stroke/transient ischemic attack rates and any bleeding event at 1-year follow-up.

2.3. Statistical Analysis

Statistical analysis was performed using R Version 3.6.3 (R Foundation for Statistical Computing, Vienna, Austria). Categorial variables are expressed as percentages and continuous variables are expressed as mean ± SD. Variables were compared using a t-test for continuous variables and a Chi-square for categorical variables. The Kaplan-Meier method was employed to calculate the probability of achieving the primary and secondary endpoints. The Cox regression model was used to calculate the hazard ratio for the primary endpoint while adjusting for potential confounders. p values < 0.05 were considered significant.

2.4. Propensity Score Matching

To ensure comparability between the LAAO and NOAC groups concerning potential confounding factors, we employed a logistic regression model to calculate the conditional propensity score. This encompassed baseline and clinical characteristics, including age, gender, hypertension, diabetes mellitus, IHD, and CHF, while the treatment group (LAAO or NOAC) served as the dependent variable. Subsequently, we conducted matching based on these conditional propensity scores and evaluated the balance using the standardized mean difference (SMD), with a threshold of SMD < 0.1 indicating a satisfactory balance.

3. Results
3.1. Study Population and Characteristics

Following propensity score matching, our cohort included 456 patients, 342 patients in the NOAC group and 114 in the LAAO group (Table 1). As for patients with CrCl ≤ 60 mL/min, our analysis included 279 patients, 217 patients in the NOAC group and 62 in the LAAO group (Table S1). All patients had paroxysmal, persistent, or permanent AF with an indication for anticoagulation according to the ESC guidelines. The mean age was 77.3 ± 10.4 years, and 59.6% were males. A sizable portion of patients had comorbidities, including hypertension (83%), diabetes (41%), ischemic heart disease (52%), congestive heart failure (37%), and a history of stroke or Transient Ischemic Attack (TIA) (39%). The mean CHA_2DS_2-VASc score was 4.02 ± 1.5, and the mean HAS-BLED score was 4.00 ± 1.3. Notably, 75% of the patients had a history of bleeding. The mean creatinine clearance was 54.4 ± 29.5 mL/min for the NOACs group and 58.3 ± 31.6 mL/min for the LAAO group (p = 0.24).

Table 1. Baseline characteristics of study participants.

	LAAO N = 114	NOACs N = 342	p
Age	77.9 ± 7.44	77.1 ± 11.2	0.409
Sex: Male	70 (61.4%)	202 (59.1%)	0.741
Hypertension	98 (86.0%)	279 (81.6%)	0.353
Diabetes Mellitus	50 (43.9%)	137 (40.1%)	0.545
Ischemic Heart Disease	62 (54.4%)	173 (50.6%)	0.552
Congestive Heart Failure	44 (38.6%)	124 (36.3%)	0.737
Ejection fraction (%)	52.5 ± 7.27	52.9 ± 11.1	0.674
Prior bleeding	85 (74.6%)	256 (74.9%)	1.000
Prior stroke or TIA	49 (43.0%)	127 (37.1%)	0.317
CrCl	58.3 ± 31.6	54.4 ± 29.5	0.243
CrCl ≤ 60 mL/min	62 (54.4%)	217 (63.5%)	0.108
CHA_2DS_2-VASc	4.17 ± 1.29	3.96 ± 1.57	0.173
CHA_2DS_2-VASc ≥ 4	83 (72.8%)	230 (67.3%)	0.322
HAS-BLED	4.14 ± 1.04	3.95 ± 1.35	0.113
HAS-BLED ≥ 4	86 (75.4%)	236 (69.0%)	0.235
Prior Aspirin treatment	49 (43.0%)	126 (36.8%)	0.291

LAAO: Left Atrial Appendage Occlusion; NOACs: Novel Oral Anticoagulants; TIA: Transient Ischemic Attack; CrCl: Creatinine Clearance, mL/min.

3.2. Primary Endpoint

The primary endpoint, all-cause 1-year mortality, occurred in 37 patients—32 (9%) from the NOAC group and 5 (4%) from the LAAO (log-rank p = 0.059). Kaplan-Meier survival curves are presented in Figure 1. There was a significant interaction between reduced renal function and treatment group for crude mortality rates: For patients with CrCl ≤ 60 mL/min, all-cause 1-year mortality occurred in 29 (13%) vs. 2 (3%) in NOAC and LAAO group, respectively (p = 0.04), and for patients with CrCl > 60 mL/min 3 (2%) vs. 3 (6%) for NOAC and LAAO group, respectively (p = 0.36) (Table S2, Figure 2).

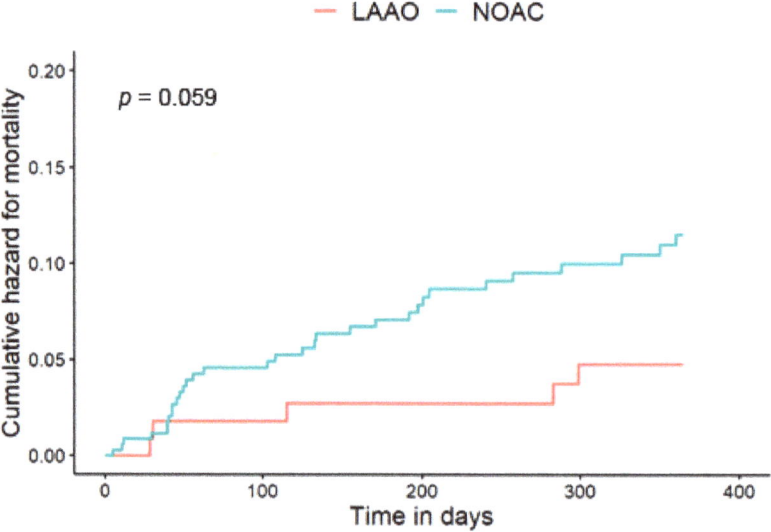

Figure 1. Kaplan-Meier curves comparing 1-year mortality of LAAO vs. NOACs. LAAO: Left Atrial Appendage Occlusion; NOACs: Novel Oral Anticoagulants.

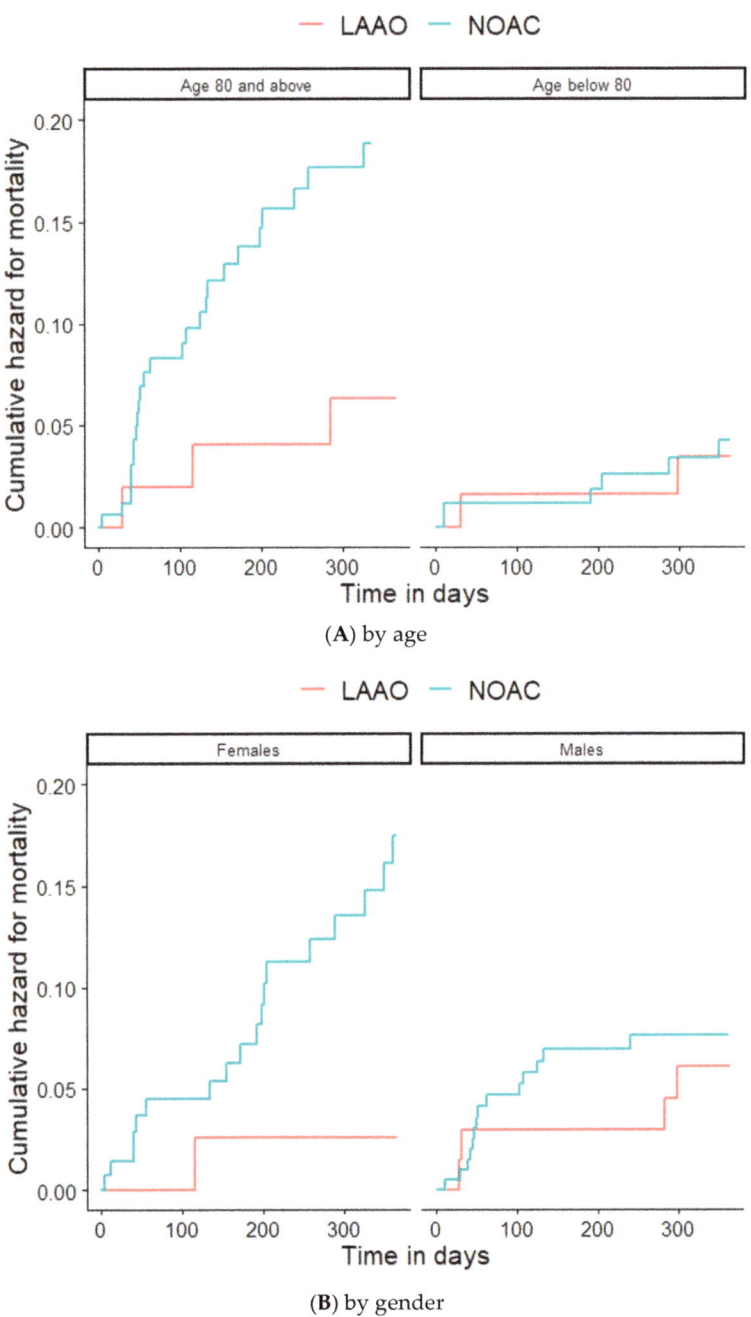

(**A**) by age

(**B**) by gender

Figure 2. *Cont.*

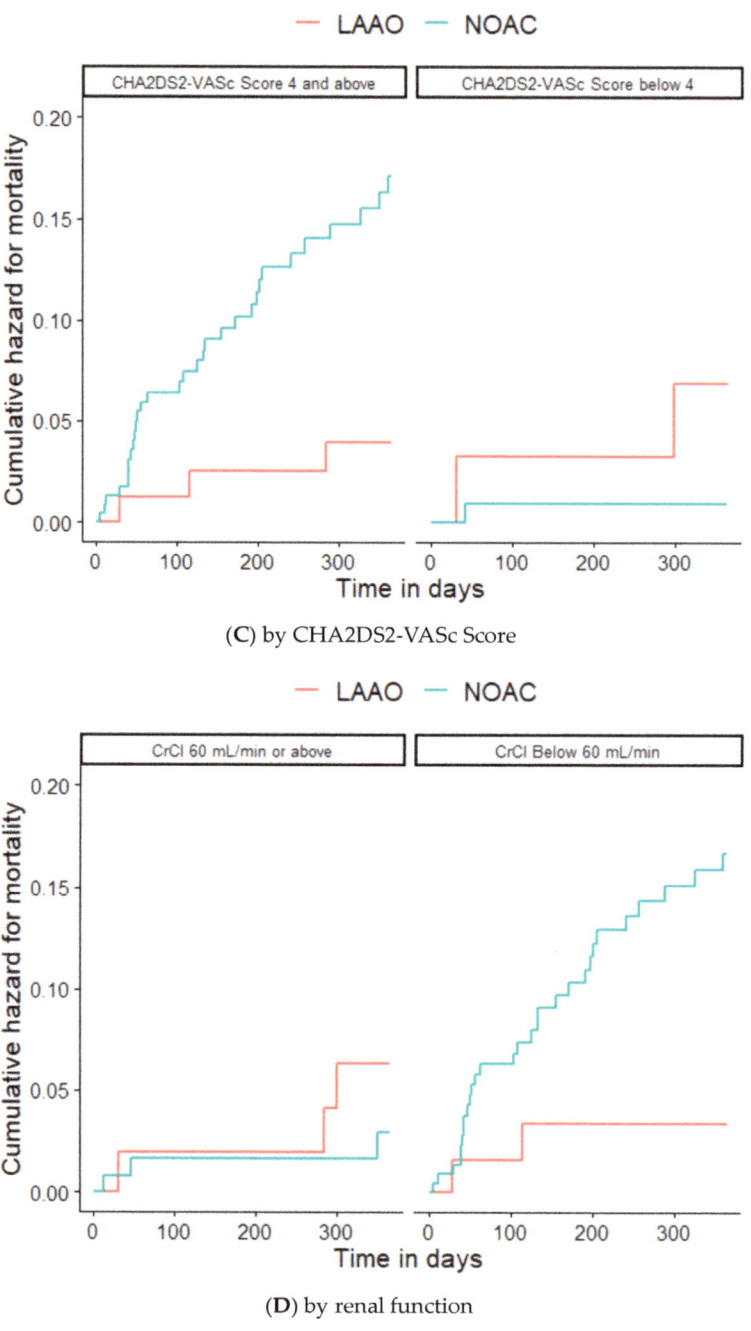

Figure 2. Kaplan-Meier curves comparing 1-year mortality of LAAO vs. NOACs by subgroups. LAAO: Left Atrial Appendage Occlusion; NOACs: Novel Oral Anticoagulant.

Table 2 shows the multivariable Cox proportional hazard analysis results by group while adjusting for age, sex, hypertension, diabetes mellitus, ischemic heart disease, heart failure, prior bleeding, prior stroke or TIA, renal function, CHA_2DS_2-VASc, and HAS-BLED scores as well as prior aspirin treatment. LAAO implantation was significantly associated with reduced risk for 1-year mortality (HR 0.38, 95%CI 0.14–0.99) compared to treatment with NOACs. Interestingly, in the subgroup analysis (Figure 3), those who underwent LAAO implantation with CrCl of <60 mL/min, CHA_2DS_2-VASc score ≥ 4, and/or those who were on a reduced NOAC dose presented with a significantly lower adjusted risk for 1-year mortality (HR 0.21, 0.23 and 0.3, respectively).

Table 2. Multivariate analysis for factors associated with 1-year mortality.

	HR (95% CI)	P
Age above 80	3.23 (1.25, 8.39)	0.016
Sex: Female	1.48 (0.51, 4.33)	0.474
Group: LAAO	0.38 (0.14, 0.99)	0.048
Congestive Heart Failure	3.87 (1.30, 11.54)	0.015
Hypertension	0.39 (0.10, 1.43)	0.154
Diabetes Mellitus	1.63 (0.52, 5.15)	0.404
Ischemic Heart Disease	1.36 (0.67, 2.77)	0.401
Ejection fraction *	0.99 (0.96, 1.02)	0.655
Prior bleeding	4.39 (0.79, 24.32)	0.09
Stroke or TIA	1.30 (0.42, 4.00)	0.645
CrCl **	0.98 (0.96, 1.00)	0.123
CHA_2DS_2-VASc	1.08 (0.48, 2.42)	0.856
HAS-BLED	0.89 (0.46, 1.73)	0.741
Aspirin treatment	1.11 (0.48, 2.58)	0.807

LAAO: Left Atrial Appendage Occlusion; TIA: Transient Ischemic Attack; CrCl: Creatinine Clearance; * Per 1 percent increment; ** Per 1 mL/min increment.

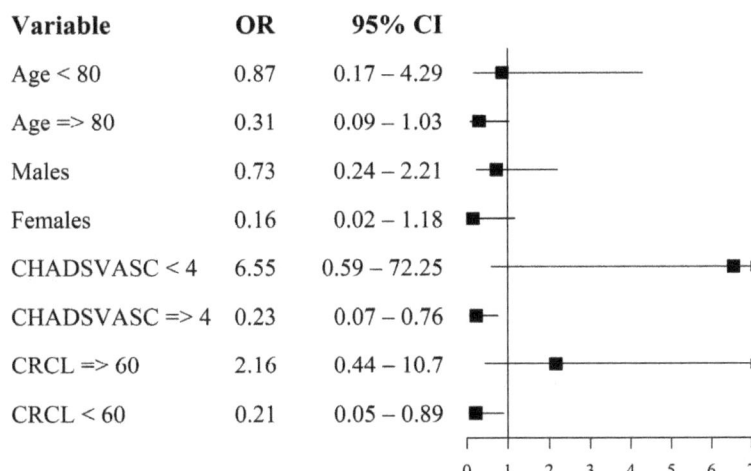

Figure 3. Subgroup analysis of factors associated with 1-year mortality for those who underwent LAAO implantation. LAAO: Left Atrial Appendage Occlusion; OR: Odds Ratio; CI: Confidence Interval; y: Years; CrCl: Creatinine Clearance.

3.3. Secondary Endpoints

At one year of follow-up, a total of 7 patients experienced stroke or TIA, 5 (1%) in the NOAC group and 2 (2%) in the LAAO group ($p = 1.00$). Likewise, major bleeding occurred in 15 patients, nine using NOACs and six in the LAAO group, without a significant between-group difference (3% vs. 5% respectively, $p = 0.22$)). Major bleeding was defined as a decrease in hemoglobin levels of 2 g/dL or more or bleeding that required a blood transfusion. Minor bleeding was defined as every bleeding which does not correspond to the definition of major bleeding. Prior bleeding was defined as any event of past major bleeding.

4. Discussion

Oral anticoagulation is recommended as the first-line therapy for preventing ischemic stroke in patients with AF and a CHA_2DS_2-VASc ≥ 1 in males and ≥ 2 in females [14]. LAAO initially emerged as an alternative therapeutic strategy for patients unable to tolerate anticoagulation or those who preferred to avoid long-term use. It proved its benefits over warfarin in several randomized controlled trials [21–23]. In the ESC guidelines, percutaneous LAAO is recommended only in patients with contraindications to anticoagulation [27,28].

In this study, which consisted of a non-direct comparison between LAAO and NOAC registries, we have demonstrated a statistically significant reduced risk for 1-year all-cause mortality in patients who underwent LAAO implantation compared to those treated with NOACs.

The results demonstrate that 1-year mortality is reduced in LAAO patients compared to NOACs, consistent with previous studies with propensity score-matched populations [24]. This finding also aligned with the PLAATO study (4.39% in the current study vs. 5.4% in PLAATO). The stroke rate in one year for the LAAO group presented in our study was comparable to the reported rate in PLAATO (1.75% vs. 1.8%, respectively). These results further support previous experience with LAAO regarding safety and efficacy in preventing stroke as reported based on the Amulet observational registry [18]. Another propensity-score matched study, which included patients with a previous ischemic stroke, compared 299 patients who underwent LAAO occlusion to 301 patients who received NOACs [29]. This analysis yielded a significantly lower (HR = 0.48) risk of the primary composite outcome of ischemic stroke, major bleeding, and all-cause mortality. The authors reported a surprisingly high rate of NOAC discontinuation of nearly 50% in 2 years. They stated that this may be one of the possible mechanisms that created differences between study arms. In a recently published real-world comparative analysis of Medicare claims data, LAAO implantation was associated with reduced risk for death, stroke, and long-term bleeding [30]. Our study correlates well with these results; however, we used a different study design—the matching ratio of 1:3 (LAAO:NOACs) vs. 1:1 in this study, and we also used the subdivision for renal failure and elderly age, whilst in the other study the gender effect was emphasized.

In this study, we performed an interaction analysis that revealed that our findings are more prominent among patients with renal failure, higher ischemic risk, and reduced NOAC dose.

4.1. Renal Failure

Renal failure is an important factor associated with increased risk for cardioembolic events and major bleeding. As such, it may play a role in the clinical decision to implant an LAAO or to medically treat eligible patients with NOACs. Lega and colleagues have demonstrated a linear relationship between the percentage of renal excretion of NOAC and the risk of major bleeding [31] while demonstrating the advantage of NOACs over warfarin. Thus, when tailoring patient-specific treatment, one should consider the inevitable course of deterioration in renal function that would eventually preclude the ability to use NOACs. Our study demonstrated a subgroup analysis with a reduced risk for 1-year all-cause mortality in patients taking reduced-dose NOACs. Under these circumstances, LAAO could be a reasonable alternative in patients with advanced kidney disease or patients with labile renal function.

There is an ongoing debate about whether treating ESRD patients with oral anticoagulants provides stroke protection over bleeding risk [32,33]. Accordingly, in the NOAC seminal studies, patients with ESRD were excluded. ESRD patients who opted to take oral anticoagulants were traditionally treated with warfarin. However, recent attempts were made to prescribe apixaban for ESRD patients, with modest evidence for the superiority of NOACs over warfarin in terms of major bleeding [34]. In our study, we had no patients with ESRD, and we cannot draw any specific conclusions. However, when considering the conflicting evidence for NOAC treatment in ESRD patients, in addition to our results in patients with CKD, LAAO could be a suitable treatment alternative in ESRD patients with NVAF.

4.2. Prior Major Bleeding

Patients with prior major bleeding were also underrepresented in the pivotal trials. The current study shows that these patients tolerated LAAO instead of NOACs (which are contraindicated in most cases) without elevated risk for rebleeding or stroke. Similarly, our study participants had higher CHA_2DS_2-VASc and HAS-BLED scores compared to the pivotal studies (4 in current study vs. 3.48, 2.1, and 2.1 in ROCKET-AF, RE-LY, and ARISTOTLE, respectively), [35] implying our study population is more similar to real-world data [36] and that our results may be generalized to other high-risk populations.

4.3. Low Dose NOACs

Patients with guideline-based indications for NOAC dose reduction are at increased risk for thrombotic and hemorrhagic complications despite being treated with anticoagulants [37]. A critical factor in determining the need for dose reduction is renal function, which also impacts the CHA_2DS_2-VASc score (indirectly by increasing risk for various cardiovascular diseases) and HAS-BLED score. The patient population with a significant advantage of using LAAO in the interaction analysis—e.g., those with an indication for reduced NOAC dose and those with increased bleeding and thrombotic risk—was the population with the most prominent cardiovascular disease burden. This phenomenon could be explained by the increased efficacy of LAAO over NOACs in stroke prevention (for example, when using a reduced NOAC dose) or by preventing unnecessary hemorrhagic phenomena among patients with labile or reduced renal function.

4.4. Limitations

Our study has several limitations. First, it is a retrospective study that utilized data from two different registries. The inclusion and exclusion criteria for the registries differ, resulting in diverse groups. We tried to mitigate this issue by applying propensity score matching. Second, as this study is based on registries, there is an inevitable loss of follow-up and inconsistency in event definition and validation. As such, we could not differentiate between major and minor bleeding. Thus, we decided to include all bleeding events regardless of severity, anatomical location, and the possible need for red blood cell transfusion. A third limitation of the study is the relatively short follow-up duration of one year. Another limitation is that we did not analyze the possible complications of LAAO implantation (such as cardiac perforation, pericardial effusion with tamponade, ischemic stroke, device embolization, and other vascular complications) [38]. In addition, we did not include information regarding the death cause of study participants. Lastly, both groups had a relatively low number of events, diminishing the power to detect other differences.

5. Conclusions

This pooled analysis of two registries demonstrated a lower risk for 1-year mortality among patients with AF who were implanted LAAO than those treated with NOACs. This result was more prominent in patients with reduced renal function. Future prospective randomized studies with larger sample sizes, ESRD and longer follow-up durations should further investigate the efficacy and adverse effects of both treatment strategies.

Supplementary Materials: The following supporting information can be downloaded at https://www.mdpi.com/article/10.3390/jcm12206693/s1. Table S1—Baseline characteristics of study participants with CrCl <= 60 mL/min, Table S2—The association between LAAO vs. NOACs and 1-year mortality – stratification by distinct groups.

Author Contributions: Data curation, S.T., A.B., I.G., N.S., E.N., R.R., M.G., V.G., I.B., R.B.; writing—original draft preparation, S.T., A.B., W.M., I.G., G.B., U.A., E.N., R.R., M.G., V.G., I.B., R.B.; writing—review and editing, S.T., A.B., W.M., I.G., G.B., U.A., E.N., R.R., M.G., V.G., I.B., R.B. All authors have read and agreed to the published version of the manuscript.

Funding: This research received no external funding.

Informed Consent Statement: Patient consent was waived due to the retrospective design of the study.

Data Availability Statement: The datasets for this study cannot be made available due to the nature of personal information they contain.

Conflicts of Interest: The authors declare no conflict of interest.

References

1. Roger, V.L.; Go, A.S.; Lloyd-Jones, D.M.; Adams, R.J.; Berry, J.D.; Brown, T.M.; Carnethon, M.R.; Dai, S.; de Simon, G.; Wylie-Rosett, J.; et al. Heart disease and stroke statistics—2011 update: A report from the American Heart Association. *Circulation* **2011**, *123*, e18–e209. [CrossRef] [PubMed]
2. Wolf, P.A.; Abbott, R.D.; Kannel, W.B. Atrial fibrillation as an independent risk factor for stroke: The Framingham Study. *Stroke* **1991**, *22*, 983–988. [CrossRef] [PubMed]
3. Coresh, J.; Selvin, E.; Stevens, L.A.; Manzi, J.; Kusek, J.W.; Eggers, P.; Van Lente, F.; Levey, A.S. Prevalence of Chronic Kidney Disease in the United States. *JAMA* **2007**, *298*, 2038–2047. [CrossRef] [PubMed]
4. Soliman, E.Z.; Prineas, R.J.; Go, A.S.; Xie, D.; Lash, J.P.; Rahman, M.; Ojo, A.; Teal, V.L.; Jensvold, N.G.; Robinson, N.L.; et al. Chronic kidney disease and prevalent atrial fibrillation: The Chronic Renal Insufficiency Cohort (CRIC). *Am. Heart J.* **2010**, *159*, 1102–1107. [CrossRef]
5. Alonso, A.; Lopez, F.L.; Matsushita, K.; Loehr, L.R.; Agarwal, S.K.; Chen, L.Y.; Soliman, E.Z.; Astor, B.; Coresh, J. Chronic kidney disease is associated with the incidence of atrial fibrillation: The Atherosclerosis Risk in Communities (ARIC) study. *Circulation* **2011**, *123*, 2946–2953. [CrossRef]
6. Baber, U.; Howard, V.J.; Halperin, J.L.; Soliman, E.Z.; Zhang, X.; McClellan, W.; Muntner, P. Association of chronic kidney disease with atrial fibrillation among adults in the United States: REasons for Geographic and Racial Differences in Stroke (REGARDS) Study. *Circ. Arrhythmia Electrophysiol.* **2011**, *4*, 26–32. [CrossRef]
7. Olesen, J.B.; Lip, G.Y.; Kamper, A.-L.; Hommel, K.; Køber, L.; Lane, D.A.; Lindhardsen, J.; Gislason, G.H.; Torp-Pedersen, C. Stroke and bleeding in atrial fibrillation with chronic kidney disease. *N. Engl. J. Med.* **2012**, *367*, 625–635. [CrossRef]
8. Hart, R.G.; Pearce, L.A.; Aguilar, M.I. Meta-analysis: Antithrombotic therapy to prevent stroke in patients who have nonvalvular atrial fibrillation. *Ann. Intern. Med.* **2007**, *146*, 857–867. [CrossRef]
9. ACTIVE Writing Group of the ACTIVE Investigators; Connolly, S.J.; Pogue, J.; Hart, R.G.; A Pfeffer, M.; Hohnloser, S.H.; Chrolavicius, S.; Yusuf, S. Clopidogrel plus aspirin versus oral anticoagulation for atrial fibrillation in the Atrial fibrillation Clopidogrel Trial with Irbesartan for prevention of Vascular Events (ACTIVE W): A randomised controlled trial. *Lancet* **2006**, *367*, 1903–1912.
10. Shameem, R.; Ansell, J. Disadvantages of VKA and requirements for novel anticoagulants. *Best Pract. Res. Clin. Haematol.* **2013**, *26*, 103–114. [CrossRef]
11. Connolly, S.J.; Eikelboom, J.; Joyner, C.; Diener, H.-C.; Hart, R.; Golitsyn, S.; Flaker, G.; Avezum, A.; Hohnloser, S.H.; Diaz, R.; et al. Apixaban in patients with atrial fibrillation. *N. Engl. J. Med.* **2011**, *364*, 806–817. [CrossRef] [PubMed]
12. Connolly, S.J.; Ezekowitz, M.D.; Yusuf, S.; Eikelboom, J.; Oldgren, J.; Parekh, A.; Pogue, J.; Reilly, P.A.; Themeles, E.; Varrone, J.; et al. Dabigatran versus warfarin in patients with atrial fibrillation. *N. Engl. J. Med.* **2009**, *361*, 1139–1151. [CrossRef] [PubMed]
13. Patel, M.R.; Mahaffey, K.W.; Garg, J.; Pan, G.; Singer, D.E.; Hacke, W.; Breithardt, G.; Halperin, J.L.; Hankey, G.J.; Piccini, J.P.; et al. Rivaroxaban versus warfarin in nonvalvular atrial fibrillation. *N. Engl. J. Med.* **2011**, *365*, 883–891. [CrossRef] [PubMed]
14. Hindricks, G.; Potpara, T.; Dagres, N.; Arbelo, E.; Bax, J.J.; Blomström-Lundqvist, C.; Boriani, G.; Castella, M.; Dan, G.-A.; Dilaveris, P.E.; et al. 2020 ESC Guidelines for the diagnosis and management of atrial fibrillation developed in collaboration with the European Association for Cardio-Thoracic Surgery (EACTS). *Eur. Heart J.* **2021**, *42*, 373–498. [CrossRef] [PubMed]
15. January, C.T.; Wann, L.S.; Alpert, J.S.; Calkins, H.; Cigarroa, J.E.; Cleveland Jr, J.C.; Yancy, C.W. 2014 AHA/ACC/HRS guideline for the management of patients with atrial fibrillation: Executive summary: A report of the American College of Cardiology/American Heart Association Task Force on practice guidelines and the Heart Rhythm Society. *Circulation* **2014**, *130*, 2071–2104. [CrossRef]
16. Freedman, B.; Potpara, T.S.; Lip, G.Y. Stroke prevention in atrial fibrillation. *Lancet* **2016**, *388*, 806–817. [CrossRef]
17. Chan, K.E.; Giugliano, R.P.; Patel, M.R.; Abramson, S.; Jardine, M.; Zhao, S.; Perkovic, V.; Maddux, F.W.; Piccini, J.P. Nonvitamin K Anticoagulant Agents in Patients With Advanced Chronic Kidney Disease or on Dialysis With AF. *J. Am. Coll. Cardiol.* **2016**, *67*, 2888–2899. [CrossRef]

18. Landmesser, U.; Tondo, C.; Camm, J.; Diener, H.C.; Paul, V.; Schmidt, B.; Hildick-Smith, D. Left atrial appendage occlusion with the AMPLATZER Amulet device: One-year follow-up from the prospective global Amulet observational registry. *EuroIntervention J. EuroPCR Collab. Work. Group Interv. Cardiol. Eur. Soc. Cardiol.* **2018**, *14*, e590–e597. [CrossRef]
19. Baman, J.R.; Mansour, M.; Heist, E.K.; Huang, D.T.; Biton, Y. Percutaneous left atrial appendage occlusion in the prevention of stroke in atrial fibrillation: A systematic review. *Heart Fail. Rev.* **2018**, *23*, 191–208. [CrossRef]
20. Ostermayer, S.H.; Reisman, M.; Kramer, P.H.; Matthews, R.V.; Gray, W.A.; Block, P.C.; Omran, H.; Bartorelli, A.L.; Della Bella, P.; Di Mario, C.; et al. Percutaneous left atrial appendage transcatheter occlusion (PLAATO System) to prevent stroke in high-risk patients with non-rheumatic atrial fibrillation: Results from the international multi-center feasibility trials. *J. Am. Coll. Cardiol.* **2005**, *46*, 9–14. [CrossRef]
21. Reddy, V.Y.; Sievert, H.; Halperin, J.; Doshi, S.K.; Buchbinder, M.; Neuzil, P.; Holmes, D. Percutaneous left atrial appendage closure vs warfarin for atrial fibrillation: A randomized clinical trial. *JAMA* **2014**, *312*, 1988–1998. [CrossRef]
22. Reddy, V.Y.; Doshi, S.K.; Kar, S.; Gibson, D.N.; Price, M.J.; Huber, K. 5-Year Outcomes after Left Atrial Appendage Closure: From the PREVAIL and PROTECT AF Trials. *J. Am. Coll. Cardiol.* **2017**, *70*, 2964–2975. [CrossRef] [PubMed]
23. Holmes, D.R.; Kar, S.; Price, M.J.; Whisenant, B.; Sievert, H.; Doshi, S.K.; Reddy, V.Y. Prospective randomized evaluation of the Watchman Left Atrial Appendage Closure device in patients with atrial fibrillation versus long-term warfarin therapy: The PREVAIL trial. *J. Am. Coll. Cardiol.* **2014**, *64*, 1–12. [CrossRef] [PubMed]
24. Nielsen-Kudsk, J.E.; Korsholm, K.; Damgaard, D.; Valentin, J.B.; Diener, H.C.; Camm, A.J.; Johnsen, S.P. Clinical Outcomes Associated with Left Atrial Appendage Occlusion versus Direct Oral Anticoagulation in Atrial Fibrillation. *Cardiovasc. Interv.* **2021**, *14*, 69–78. [CrossRef] [PubMed]
25. Whitlock, R.P.; Belley-Cote, E.P.; Paparella, D.; Healey, J.S.; Brady, K.; Sharma, M.; Reents, W.; Budera, P.; Baddour, A.J.; Fila, P.; et al. Left Atrial Appendage Occlusion during Cardiac Surgery to Prevent Stroke. *N. Engl. J. Med.* **2021**, *384*, 2081–2091. [CrossRef]
26. Osmancik, P.; Herman, D.; Neuzil, P.; Hala, P.; Taborsky, M.; Kala, P.; Poloczek, M.; Stasek, J.; Haman, L.; Branny, M.; et al. Left Atrial Appendage Closure Versus Direct Oral Anticoagulants in High-Risk Patients With Atrial Fibrillation. *J. Am. Coll. Cardiol.* **2020**, *75*, 3122–3135. [CrossRef]
27. Saw, J.; Holmes, D.R.; Cavalcante, J.L.; Freeman, J.V.; Goldsweig, A.M.; Kavinsky, C.J.; Moussa, I.D.; Munger, T.M.; Price, M.J.; Reisman, M.; et al. SCAI/HRS Expert Consensus Statement on Transcatheter Left Atrial Appendage Closure. *JACC: Cardiovasc. Interv.* **2023**, *16*, 1384–1400.
28. Glikson, M.; Wolff, R.; Hindricks, G.; Mandrola, J.; Camm, A.J.; Lip, G.Y.H.; Fauchier, L.; Betts, T.R.; Lewalter, T.; Saw, J.; et al. EHRA/EAPCI expert consensus statement on catheter-based left atrial appendage occlusion—An update. *Europace* **2020**, *22*, 184. [CrossRef]
29. Korsholm, K.; Valentin, J.B.; Damgaard, D.; Diener, H.-C.; Camm, A.J.; Landmesser, U.; Hildick-Smith, D.; Johnsen, S.P.; Nielsen-Kudsk, J.E. Clinical outcomes of left atrial appendage occlusion versus direct oral anticoagulation in patients with atrial fibrillation and prior ischemic stroke: A propensity-score matched study. *Int. J. Cardiol.* **2022**, *363*, 56–63. [CrossRef]
30. Zeitler, E.P.; Kearing, S.; Coylewright, M.; Nair, D.; Hsu, J.C.; Darden, D.; O'malley, A.J.; Russo, A.M.; Al-Khatib, S.M. Comparative Effectiveness of Left Atrial Appendage Occlusion Versus Oral Anticoagulation by Sex. *Circulation* **2023**, *147*, 586–596. [CrossRef]
31. Lega, J.; Bertoletti, L.; Gremillet, C.; Boissier, C.; Mismetti, P.; Laporte, S. Consistency of safety profile of new oral anticoagulants in patients with renal failure. *J. Thromb. Haemost.* **2014**, *12*, 337–343. [CrossRef] [PubMed]
32. Chan, K.E.; Lazarus, J.M.; Thadhani, R.; Hakim, R.M. Anticoagulant and Antiplatelet Usage Associates with Mortality among Hemodialysis Patients. *J. Am. Soc. Nephrol.* **2009**, *20*, 872–881. [CrossRef] [PubMed]
33. Van Der Meersch, H.; De Bacquer, D.; De Vriese, A.S. Vitamin K antagonists for stroke prevention in hemodialysis patients with atrial fibrillation: A systematic review and meta-analysis. *Am. Heart J.* **2017**, *184*, 37–46. [CrossRef] [PubMed]
34. Siontis, K.C.; Zhang, X.; Eckard, A.; Bhave, N.; Schaubel, D.E.; He, K.; Nallamothu, B.K. Outcomes Associated with Apixaban use in Patients with End-Stage Kidney Disease and Atrial Fibrillation in the United States. *Circulation* **2018**, *138*, 1519–1529. [CrossRef] [PubMed]
35. Lee, S.; Monz, B.U.; Clemens, A.; Brueckmann, M.; Lip, G.Y.H. Representativeness of the dabigatran, apixaban and rivaroxaban clinical trial populations to real-world atrial fibrillation patients in the United Kingdom: A cross-sectional analysis using the General Practice Research Database. *BMJ Open* **2012**, *2*, e001768. [CrossRef]
36. Bertaglia, E.; Anselmino, M.; Zorzi, A.; Russo, V.; Toso, E.; Peruzza, F.; Rapacciuolo, A.; Migliore, F.; Gaita, F.; Cucchini, U.; et al. NOACs and atrial fibrillation: Incidence and predictors of left atrial thrombus in the real world. *Int. J. Cardiol.* **2017**, *249*, 179–183. [CrossRef]
37. Wang, K.-L.; Lopes, R.D.; Patel, M.R.; Büller, H.R.; Tan, D.S.-Y.; Chiang, C.-E.; Giugliano, R.P. Efficacy and safety of reduced-dose non-vitamin K antagonist oral anticoagulants in patients with atrial fibrillation: A meta-analysis of randomized controlled trials. *Eur. Heart J.* **2018**, *40*, 1492–1500. [CrossRef]
38. Sharma, S.P.; Park, P.; Lakkireddy, D. Left Atrial Appendages Occlusion: Current Status and Prospective. *Korean Circ. J.* **2018**, *48*, 692–704. [CrossRef]

Disclaimer/Publisher's Note: The statements, opinions and data contained in all publications are solely those of the individual author(s) and contributor(s) and not of MDPI and/or the editor(s). MDPI and/or the editor(s) disclaim responsibility for any injury to people or property resulting from any ideas, methods, instructions or products referred to in the content.

MDPI
St. Alban-Anlage 66
4052 Basel
Switzerland
www.mdpi.com

Journal of Clinical Medicine Editorial Office
E-mail: jcm@mdpi.com
www.mdpi.com/journal/jcm

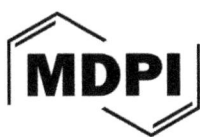

Disclaimer/Publisher's Note: The statements, opinions and data contained in all publications are solely those of the individual author(s) and contributor(s) and not of MDPI and/or the editor(s). MDPI and/or the editor(s) disclaim responsibility for any injury to people or property resulting from any ideas, methods, instructions or products referred to in the content.